STANDARDIZING MEDICATION LABELS

Confusing Patients Less

Workshop Summary

Lyla M. Hernandez, *Rapporteur*

Roundtable on Health Literacy

Board on Population Health and Public Health Practice

INSTITUTE OF MEDICINE
OF THE NATIONAL ACADEMIES

THE NATIONAL ACADEMIES PRESS
Washington, D.C.
www.nap.edu

THE NATIONAL ACADEMIES PRESS   500 Fifth Street, N.W.   Washington, DC 20001

NOTICE: The project that is the subject of this report was approved by the Governing Board of the National Research Council, whose members are drawn from the councils of the National Academy of Sciences, the National Academy of Engineering, and the Institute of Medicine. The members of the committee responsible for the report were chosen for their special competences and with regard for appropriate balance.

This project was supported by contracts between the National Academy of Sciences and the UnitedHealth Group (unnumbered award); Academy for Educational Development (unnumbered award); Kaiser Permanente (unnumbered award); American Academy of Family Physicians (unnumbered award); Affinity Health Plan (unnumbered award); Merck & Co., Inc. (unnumbered award); Pfizer Institute (unnumbered award); Department of Health and Human Services (N01-OD-4-2139, TO#148); and Glaxo Smith Kline (G050002912). Any opinions, findings, conclusions, or recommendations expressed in this publication are those of the author(s) and do not necessarily reflect the view of the organizations or agencies that provided support for this project.

This summary is based on the proceedings of a workshop that was sponsored by the Roundtable on Health Literacy. It is prepared in the form of a workshop summary by and in the name of the rapporteur as an individually authored document.

International Standard Book Number-13:   978-0-309-11529-2
International Standard Book Number-10:   0-309-11529-9

Additional copies of this report are available from the National Academies Press, 500 Fifth Street, N.W., Lockbox 285, Washington, DC 20055; (800) 624-6242 or (202) 334-3313 (in the Washington metropolitan area); Internet, http://www.nap.edu.

For more information about the Institute of Medicine, visit the IOM home page at **www.iom.edu.**

Printed in the United States of America

The serpent has been a symbol of long life, healing, and knowledge among almost all cultures and religions since the beginning of recorded history. The serpent adopted as a logotype by the Institute of Medicine is a relief carving from ancient Greece, now held by the Staatliche Museen in Berlin.

Suggested citation: IOM (Institute of Medicine). 2008. Standardizing medication labels: Confusing patients less, workshop summary. Washington, DC: The National Academies Press.

"Knowing is not enough; we must apply.
Willing is not enough; we must do."
—Goethe

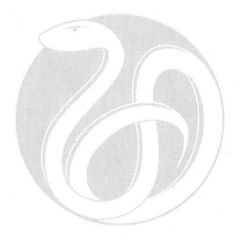

INSTITUTE OF MEDICINE
OF THE NATIONAL ACADEMIES

Advising the Nation. Improving Health.

THE NATIONAL ACADEMIES
Advisers to the Nation on Science, Engineering, and Medicine

The **National Academy of Sciences** is a private, nonprofit, self-perpetuating society of distinguished scholars engaged in scientific and engineering research, dedicated to the furtherance of science and technology and to their use for the general welfare. Upon the authority of the charter granted to it by the Congress in 1863, the Academy has a mandate that requires it to advise the federal government on scientific and technical matters. Dr. Ralph J. Cicerone is president of the National Academy of Sciences.

The **National Academy of Engineering** was established in 1964, under the charter of the National Academy of Sciences, as a parallel organization of outstanding engineers. It is autonomous in its administration and in the selection of its members, sharing with the National Academy of Sciences the responsibility for advising the federal government. The National Academy of Engineering also sponsors engineering programs aimed at meeting national needs, encourages education and research, and recognizes the superior achievements of engineers. Dr. Charles M. Vest is president of the National Academy of Engineering.

The **Institute of Medicine** was established in 1970 by the National Academy of Sciences to secure the services of eminent members of appropriate professions in the examination of policy matters pertaining to the health of the public. The Institute acts under the responsibility given to the National Academy of Sciences by its congressional charter to be an adviser to the federal government and, upon its own initiative, to identify issues of medical care, research, and education. Dr. Harvey V. Fineberg is president of the Institute of Medicine.

The **National Research Council** was organized by the National Academy of Sciences in 1916 to associate the broad community of science and technology with the Academy's purposes of furthering knowledge and advising the federal government. Functioning in accordance with general policies determined by the Academy, the Council has become the principal operating agency of both the National Academy of Sciences and the National Academy of Engineering in providing services to the government, the public, and the scientific and engineering communities. The Council is administered jointly by both Academies and the Institute of Medicine. Dr. Ralph J. Cicerone and Dr. Charles M. Vest are chair and vice chair, respectively, of the National Research Council.

www.national-academies.org

MEMBERS OF THE PLANNING GROUP FOR THE WORKSHOP ON CHANGING PRESCRIPTION MEDICATION USE CONTAINER INSTRUCTIONS TO IMPROVE HEALTH LITERACY AND MEDICATION SAFETY

CAROLYN COCOTAS, R.T., M.P.A., Director, Affinity Health Plan

JEAN KRAUSE, Executive Vice President and CEO, American College of Physicians Foundation

RUTH PARKER, M.D., Associate Professor of Medicine, Emory University School of Medicine

ANDY STERGACHIS, Ph.D., R.Ph., Professor of Epidemiology, University of Washington

DONNA SWEET, M.D., Director of Internal Medicine Education, Via Christi Regional Medical Center–St. Francis

CAROL TEUTSCH, M.D., Director of Medical Services, Merck & Co.

SABRA WOOLLEY, Ph.D., Program Director, Health Communication and Informatics Branch, National Cancer Institute

---

IOM planning committees are solely responsible for organizing the workshop, identifying topics, and choosing speakers. The responsibility for the published workshop summary rests with the workshop rapporteur and the institution.

MEMBERS OF THE ROUNDTABLE ON HEALTH LITERACY

ANTRONETTE YANCEY, M.D., M.P.H., Associate Professor of
Health Services and Director, Doctorate in Public Health Program,
University of California, School of Public Health, Los Angeles

Staff

ROSE MARIE MARTINEZ, Sc.D., Director, Board on Population
Health and Public Health Practice
LYLA M. HERNANDEZ, M.P.H., Senior Program Officer
HOPE R. HARE, M.F.A., Administrative Assistant
TIA CARTER, Senior Project Assistant

IOM forums and roundtables do not issue, review, or approve individual documents. The responsibility for the published workshop summary rests with the workshop rapporteur and the institution.

Reviewers

This report has been reviewed in draft form by individuals chosen for their diverse perspectives and technical expertise, in accordance with procedures approved by the National Research Council's Report Review Committee. The purpose of this independent review is to provide candid and critical comments that will assist the institution in making its published report as sound as possible and to ensure that the report meets institutional standards for objectivity, evidence, and responsiveness to the study charge. The review comments and draft manuscript remain confidential to protect the integrity of the deliberative process. We wish to thank the following individuals for their review of this report:

Diane D. Cousins, R.Ph., United States Pharmacopeia Standards Division, Department of Healthcare Quality & Information
Susan Cummins, M.D., Food and Drug Administration, Center for Drug Evaluation and Research, U.S. Department of Health and Human Services
Hugh Tilson, M.D., Ph.D., Public Health Leadership Program, University of North Carolina School of Public Health
Winston F. Wong, M.D., M.S., Disparities Improvement and Quality Initiatives, Kaiser Permanente, National Program Office

Although the reviewers listed above have provided many constructive comments and suggestions, they were not asked to endorse a final draft of the report before its release. The review of this report was overseen by **Harold J. Fallon, M.D.,** School of Medicine, University of Alabama at Birmingham. Appointed by the Institute of Medicine, he was responsible for making certain that an independent examination of this report was carried out in accordance with institutional procedures and that all review comments were carefully considered. Responsibility for the final content of this report rests entirely with the author and the institution.

Acknowledgments

Without the support of the sponsors of the Institute of Medicine Roundtable on Health Literacy, it would not have been possible to plan and conduct the workshop on standardizing medication labels that this report summarizes. Sponsors from the Department of Health and Human Services are the Centers for Medicare and Medicaid Services, the Health Resources and Services Administration, the Office of Disease Prevention and Health Promotion, and the National Cancer Institute. Non-federal sponsorship is provided by the Academy for Education Development, Affinity Health Plan, the American Academy of Family Physicians Foundation, GlaxoSmithKline, Kaiser Permanente, Merck and Co., Inc., and Pfizer, Inc.

The Roundtable is especially grateful to UnitedHealth Group, which provided funds specifically for this workshop. The American College of Physicians Foundation commissioned a thoughtful white paper, Improving Prescription Drug Container Labeling in the United States: A Health Literacy and Medication Safety Initiative, which provided an important base of information for workshop participants.

The Roundtable wishes to express its gratitude to the four expert speakers whose presentations provided the background for the issues on medication labeling: Dan Budnitz, Terry C. Davis, Michael Wolf, and Alastair Wood. Additional thanks go to Alastair Wood, who developed and presented a proposal for standardization of medication labels that energized discussion. Reactions to these presentations were provided by the following distinguished individuals: Cindy Brach, William Bullman,

Vanessa Cajina, William Dolan, Merrill J. Egorin, William Ellis, Alan Goldhammer, Susan Johnson, Mary Ann F. Kirkpatrick, Gerald McEvoy, Nancy Ostrove, Virginia Torrise, Darren Townzen, Linda Weiss, Roger Williams, Albert Wu, and Mara Youdelman.

The Roundtable wishes to thank the planning committee members for their hard work in putting together an excellent workshop agenda. Members of the planning committee are Carolyn Cocotas, Jean Krause, Rose Marie Martinez, Ruth Parker, Andy Stergachis, Donna Sweet, Carol Teutsch, and Sabra Woolley. Thanks also go to George Isham for moderating the entire workshop.

Contents

xiii

TABLES

FIGURES

1

Introduction

Medications are an important component of health care, but each year their misuse results in over a million adverse drug events (ADEs)[1] (IOM, 2007) that lead to office and emergency room visits as well as hospitalizations and, in some cases, death. As a patient's most tangible source of information about what drug has been prescribed and how that drug is to be taken, the label on a container of prescription medication is a crucial line of defense against such ADEs, yet according to Michael Wolf of Northwestern University's Feinberg School of Medicine, 46 percent of patients across all literacy levels misunderstand one or more dosage instructions and 54 percent misunderstand one or more auxiliary warnings that accompany those medications. To examine what is known about how medication container labeling affects patient safety and to discuss approaches to addressing identified problems, the Institute of Medicine Roundtable on Health Literacy organized a workshop, Changing Prescription Medication Use Container Instructions to Improve Health Literacy and Medication Safety, which was held on October 12, 2007.[2]

---

[1]Adverse drug events are defined as harm or injury occurring from legal medication use and exclude intentional drug abuse or intentional self-harm or suicide attempts.

[2]The planning committee's role was limited to planning the workshop, and the workshop summary has been prepared by the workshop rapporteur as a factual summary of what occurred at the workshop.

THE WORKSHOP AGENDA

The first part of the workshop consisted of four presentations designed to (1) describe problems in ambulatory care drug safety; (2) examine the role of health literacy in patient care; (3) present findings from the American College of Physicians Foundation white paper on drug labeling; and (4) offer a proposal for standardization of drug labeling. The second part of the conference consisted of reactions to the four initial presentations by representatives from federal agencies, the pharmacy field, and other stakeholders, as well as discussion of what it would take to move towards standardization in drug labeling instructions. The workshop was moderated by George Isham, M.D., M.S., chair of the IOM Roundtable on Health Literacy.

2

Presentations

DRUG SAFETY IN AMBULATORY CARE

Dan Budnitz, M.D., M.P.H.
Centers for Disease Control and Prevention

Adverse drug events (ADEs) are responsible for 3.6 million office visits a year, 700,000 emergency room visits, and 117,000 hospitalizations, according to Dan Budnitz at the Centers for Disease Control and Prevention (Budnitz et al., 2006; Zhan et al., 2005). Dosing mistakes appear to cause a disproportionate number of the most severe ADEs, with over half of the hospitalizations caused by unintended overdoses or supratherapeutic drug levels. An examination of emergency visits for ADEs shows that patient age is a risk factor, with those ages under 5 and over 65 at greater risk than others.

Interventions to prevent ADEs have been implemented primarily in hospitals and have focused on preventing medication errors[1] through computerization and systems changes. In the hospital environment, health professionals prescribe and monitor the use of medications and have extensive support systems.

In the ambulatory setting, however, patients play a key role in drug safety since medications may be prescribed by a health professional or may be self-prescribed by the patient, and patients or other laypersons

---

[1]Medication error is defined as any preventable event that may lead to inappropriate medication use or patient harm.

are the ones responsible for administering, storing, and monitoring the use of medications. Support systems for the patient are minimal in the ambulatory setting, and in some instances the medication container label may be the only source of information for the patient.

Although medication injuries often result from a complex interaction of agent, host, and environment, the most appropriate basis for identifying safety interventions may be patient-focused approaches such as those used in the injury-prevention field. The first step in an injury-prevention approach uses a heuristic called a phase–factor matrix (originally developed by Haddon) (Figure 2-1) to identify plausible interventions.

In this matrix the three phases of the injury process appear in the left-hand column: pre-event, event (or the injury), and post-event. Across the top of the matrix are the three entities among which the interactions traditionally occur to cause an injury or disease: the host or patient, the agent or drug, and the environment. When the phase–factor matrix was used to identify interventions for ADEs from Warfarin, the first two environmental changes identified were standardized naming and dosing conventions and improved medication label readability for patients (Budnitz and Layde, 2007).

Once interventions are identified, the second step in the injury-prevention approach is to consider implementation strategies since different strategies require different actions on the part of individuals, stakeholders, and society, and each strategy has different strengths, weaknesses, costs, and feasibility. Strategies include education, enforcement (e.g., laws mandating use of seat belts), and engineering (e.g., better medication label design). Injury-prevention strategies are typically classified as

Factor \ Phase	Host (Patient)	Agent (Drug)	Environment
Pre-Event			
Event			
Post-Event			

FIGURE 2-1 Phase–factor matrix for identifying plausible intervention. SOURCE: Budnitz (2007).

either active or passive. Active approaches require action on the part of an individual (e.g., actively disposing of needles and sharps containers), whereas passive approaches do not require action by the individual (e.g., the use of needleless IV connectors throughout a hospital). Typically passive approaches are more sustainable. Finally, it is critical to evaluate the impact of these interventions.

Budnitz concluded that drug safety for ambulatory patients is an important public health problem that offers an opportunity to develop and implement patient-centered drug safety measures such as standardized naming and dosing instructions.

THE ROLE OF HEALTH LITERACY IN PATIENT CARE

Terry C. Davis, Ph.D.
Louisiana State University Health Sciences Center

Ninety million Americans have trouble understanding and acting on health information, reported Terry Davis of the Louisiana State University Health Sciences Center. How well people understand medication container labels is a function of both the clarity of the labels and the degree of people's health literacy. When there is a gap between the complexity of health information and a person's ability to understand and use that information, misunderstandings occur. The National Assessment of Health Literacy identifies four levels of health literacy: below basic, basic, intermediate, and proficient. Only two-thirds of those who fall into the below basic level are even able to circle the date on a doctor's appointment slip.

In 2003, the National Assessment of Health Literacy found that only 12 percent of adults scored in the proficient category. Twenty-two percent of Medicare beneficiaries scored in the basic range, Davis observed, yet the elderly, on average, fill 27 prescriptions a year and see 8 different physicians. Fifty-three percent of high school graduates scored in the very low intermediate range. Only two-thirds of those in the intermediate range—53 percent of the population—are able to determine what time to take a prescription medicine based on the label. Patients are not taught to read labels, yet it is assumed that patients who receive medicines will be able to understand instructions for proper use (NAAL, 2005).

Medication errors are the most common medical mistake, said Davis. While labeling instructions and auxiliary warnings appear simple, according to a study of 395 patients by Davis and colleagues (2007), they are often misunderstood. For example, the auxiliary label instructing "take with food" (see Figure 2-2) appears straightforward. It is written at a first-grade level. Yet 16 percent of patients did not understand this label.

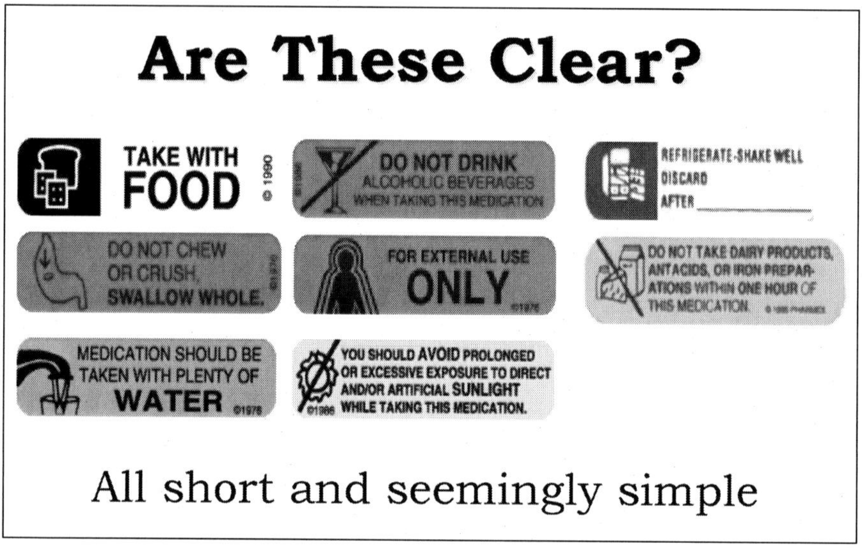

FIGURE 2-2 Auxiliary warning labels.
SOURCE: Davis et al. (2007).

Another auxiliary label in Figure 2-2 above states "medication should be taken with plenty of water." However, the label does not say how much is plenty; only 59 percent of patients understood that label. Furthermore, unfamiliar, multistep instructions such as "do not take dairy products, antacids, or iron preparations within one hour of this medication" are even more confusing. Only 8 percent understood this instruction (Davis et al., 2007).

In response to a question, Wolf observed that the problem of auxiliary warning labels is compounded when the patient is not fluent in English. Of the 114 auxiliary labels, few have been translated into Spanish and none into other languages. The Walgreen Company is implementing a program that provides translations of medication information in several languages, but the effectiveness of the program has not yet been evaluated.

Using icons does not necessarily make instructions clearer, Davis said. For example, in Figure 2-2 the warning label stating "do not chew or crush, swallow whole" includes an icon intended to show a whole pill heading into the stomach, but the meaning of the icon was not clear. Some patients interpreted the icon to mean "someone swallowed a nickel," while others thought it indicated "indigestion" or "a bladder" or said that "it looks like a ghost—Casper." Nor did adding words to the icon help clarify instructions. Various patients interpreted the words to mean "chew pill and crush before swallowing," "chew it up so it will dissolve," "don't swallow whole or you might choke," and "just for your stomach" (Davis et al., 2007).

In a study by Davis and colleagues (2006a), patients were given five pill bottles with instructions on the label. They were then asked how they would take the medication. Nearly half the patients (46 percent) did not understand at least one of the labels, and even among those with adequate literacy, more than a third (38 percent) missed at least one of the labels. When asked specifically how many pills they would take if the instructions (written at a sixth-grade level) were "take two tablets by mouth twice daily," 71 percent said they would take two pills two times a day but only about a third could demonstrate what that meant—that is, actually count out four pills.

The study authors then measured comprehension of the instructions "take two pills in the morning and two pills in the evening" (seventh-grade level writing), and "take two pills by mouth at 8:00 a.m. and two pills at 6:00 p.m." (eighth-grade level writing). The results, shown in Figure 2-3, demonstrate that the instructions written at the higher grade levels—seventh and eighth—were actually understood by more people than those written at the sixth-grade level. The comprehension also increased, despite the increased reading level, because instructions were more precise. Davis also commented that the problem of misunderstand-

Comprehension of Glyburide Instructions by Literacy		
Rx Dose Instructions	**Literacy**	
	High	**Low**
Take 2 tablets by mouth twice daily. (6th grade level)	71	33*
Take 2 pills in the morning and 2 pills in the evening. (7th grade level)	92	76[‡]
Take 2 pills by mouth at 8 am and 2 pills at 6 pm. (8th grade level)	90	76
*p < 0.001, ‡p < 0.01		

FIGURE 2-3 Readability does not equal clarity.
SOURCE: Davis et al. (2007).

ing medication labels is not confined to the United States, but is rather a worldwide problem.

While many might assume that misunderstanding medication label instructions is confined to those with low health literacy, in fact the problem is more widespread. As a patient who underwent mitral valve surgery herself, Davis reported experiencing several problems in understanding, even though she is a professor of medicine. First, instructions were not clear for the medications she was given. For example, Davis was given the prescription medication Coumadin. However, the Coumadin bottles had different instructions on them. One label read "take 1 and ½ tabs (7.5 mg) by mouth Tues, Thurs, Sat, and Sun and 2 tabs (10 mg) Mon, Wed, Fri," while another labeled bottle of Coumadin stated "take one (1) tablet by mouth or as directed." In addition to the confusing medication instructions, the drug names of numerous medications were strange and not useful, Davis's provider was unaware that she was going too fast with unfamiliar routine discharge instructions, and Davis was too overwhelmed and embarrassed to ask all the questions that needed to be asked.

While medication container labels appear simple, they are not necessarily clear and mistakes are common. There is a tremendous amount of variability in the wording of the instructions, in the icons used, and in the colors of auxiliary medication labels. An ability to read the label does not guarantee correct interpretation. Furthermore, mistakes are more likely as the number of medications a patient is taking increases, and the variability of dosing instructions is a source of confusion. Instructions need to be tested with patients, Davis concluded.

THE AMERICAN COLLEGE OF PHYSICIANS FOUNDATION WHITE PAPER ON DRUG LABELING: FINDINGS

Michael Wolf, Ph.D., M.P.H.
Feinberg School of Medicine, Northwestern University

The charge to the Medication Labeling Technical Advisory Board of the American College of Physicians (ACP) Foundation was to examine the current evidence about patients' ability to understand and successfully use medication labels, to identify barriers to labeling reform, and to engage stakeholders in planning how to improve medication labels for patients.

Ideally, when a drug is prescribed for a patient, the prescribing physician provides adequate counseling about the drug's purpose and how to administer it. Several studies demonstrate, however, that there is actually little communication with patients at the point of prescribing new medicines and that patients often leave the doctor's office with very little information about what drugs they are taking, what they are used for, and how they should be taken. An audience member questioned whether physicians had time available for adequate counseling, given the constraints of practice, especially in poorer communities. Wolf responded that effective counseling can be provided in the limited time available as demonstrated with studies on such topics as colon cancer screening and other preventive services. However, such effective counseling requires provider training that, to date, has not been undertaken. Wolf pointed out that patients who have been given an explanation of why they are taking a drug take the drug most effectively.

Few patients are given any sort of printed material about their medications other than the written prescription forms. Those forms are intended primarily for the purpose of communicating with the pharmacist and usually contain Latin abbreviations that, while useful to the pharmacist, are of little value to patients. Ideally, when the patient obtains medication from the pharmacist, the pharmacist will counsel the patient, answering questions and making sure that the patient understands how to use the drug. Studies show, however, that there is little such verbal communication. The patient receives his or her medication in a bag with accompanying written material such as the consumer medication information (CMI)[2] sheet and appropriate package inserts. These documents are of great length and are difficult to comprehend. One study appearing in the 2006 issue of Patient Education Counseling showed that less than a third of patients attend to information stapled to the bag and that patients frequently discard these sheets, especially patients with low literacy skills (Wolf et al., 2006b).

Because there is so little actual communication between the prescribing physician and the patient and between the pharmacist and the patient, the patient's primary guide for medication use ends up being the medication container label. Patients with high health literacy may turn to informal sources such as the Food and Drug Administration (FDA) website or the *AARP Guide to Pills*; however, those with low literacy skills are less likely to seek out health information beyond what they are told by their primary care providers.

Studies dating back to the late 1980s have found high rates of patient misunderstanding of both dose instructions and auxiliary warnings on medication labels. For example, a recent study examined patients' understanding of label instructions and found that 46 percent of all patients misunderstood one or more dosage instructions. Furthermore, fewer than 10 percent of patients actually read auxiliary warning labels, and of those, 54 percent misunderstood one or more auxiliary warnings (Davis et al.,

---

[2]CMI is written information about prescription drugs developed by organizations or individuals other than a drug's manufacturer that is intended for distribution to consumers at the time the drug is dispensed (FDA, 2006).

2006a; Wolf et al., 2006a). It is also the case that older adults and those taking multiple medication regimens are at significantly greater risk for misunderstanding and misuse of medications.

Therefore, finding number one of the ACP Foundation white paper is that "Inadequate patient understanding of prescription dosing instructions and warnings is prevalent and a significant safety concern." (See Appendix C.)

In addition to the problem of misunderstanding of label instructions, variability in medication labels leads to another problem. For prescription medications the FDA requires that certain information appear on the drug container label: drug name, pharmacy name and address, serial/lot number of the prescription, prescribing physician name, patient name, and instructions for use. The assumption is that prescription medications are used under the guidance of a physician (the learned intermediary) who will be communicating necessary information regarding use. Beyond the FDA requirements, state boards of pharmacy are responsible for establishing further standards. In response to such regulations, national pharmacy chains have developed 31 different label styles, resulting in variability in the clarity and complexity of medication use instructions (ACPF, 2007).

Finding number two of the white paper is that "Lack of universal standards and regulations for medication labeling is a root cause for medication error."

The ACP Foundation white paper concludes that there is value in attempting to improve prescription labels since they are the most tangible source of information patients receive, they are brief, and they are repeatedly used. The question then is, How can the medication label be improved?

Wolf observed that there are three decades of research and hundreds of studies that have examined variability in medication labels and how drug labels can be improved. For example, a study appearing in the September 2007 issue of the *Archives of Internal Medicine* (Shrank et al., 2007) examined variability in label content and format when identical prescriptions were dispensed at 85 different pharmacies in four cities in the United States. The study found that the current labeling system emphasized information important to the provider (e.g., pharmacy logo and prescription number) rather than information that supports understanding and use of the medication. These studies point to the need for standards that address what content should be on the drug label, the formatting and font size to use, the best types of icons to support auxiliary instructions, how better to present dosage instructions on the label, and how to be more explicit and concise when telling people how to take their medicine.

Finding number three of the ACP Foundation white paper states that "An evidence-based set of practices should guide all label content and format." The existing evidence base for label standards supports the following practices:

1. Use explicit text to describe dosage and interval in instructions.
2. Use a recognizable visual aid to convey dosage and use instructions.
3. Simplify language, avoiding unfamiliar words and medical jargon.
4. When possible, include indication for use.
5. Include distinguishable front and back sides to the label.
6. Organize the label in a patient-centered manner.
7. Improve typography: use larger, sans serif font.
8. When applicable, use numeric instead of alphabetic characters.
9. Use typographic cues (bolding and highlighting) for patient content only.
10. Use horizontal text only.
11. Use a standard icon system for signaling and organizing.

Beyond the content and format, one of the most important things on the prescription drug label is the "sig line" or dosage instruction. This information also causes the most difficulties. It is the information that patients are looking for, yet there are high levels of variability in how such information is presented. Furthermore, while instructions are seemingly simple, they are often unclear and require patient interpretation. For example, health literacy best practices indicated that the instruction "take 2 tablets by mouth twice daily" would be clearer if it read "take 2 tables in the morning and 2 tablets at bedtime" (Davis et al., 2006b).

Finding number four of the white paper states that "Instructions for use on the container label are especially important for patients and should be written in the most clear, concise manner. Language should be standardized to improve patient understanding for safe and effective use."

While the drug label is of primary importance, it is only one part of a larger system of written material on medication use that includes such things as patient information leaflets, package inserts, and CMI sheets. These materials do not meet acceptable standards for the design of health information, Wolf observed. Additionally, they are not well integrated into the pharmacy dispensing system. For example, in the study of 85 pharmacies mentioned above (Shrank et al., 2007), one of the drugs prescribed required an FDA-approved and mandated medication guide to be distributed with the prescriptions. Of the 85 pharmacies, none distributed the medication guide. Why not? In order to distribute the FDA-mandated medication guide, the pharmacist has to identify the medication as one that requires a guide, then has to find a copy of the guide. These guides are not integrated into the pharmacy system. However, pharmacy software systems automatically generate a patient information leaflet to accompany each prescription.

Finding number five of the white paper states that "Drug labeling should be viewed as an integrated system of patient information. Improvements are needed beyond the container label, and other sources of consumer medication information should be targeted."

Medication labeling changes cannot and should not replace provider counseling. The physician is the learned intermediary, that is, the person who is legally responsible for communicating important information about prescription drugs to patients. Moreover, health communication research has shown that physicians are the most important and trusted source of health information. Pharmacists also have a mandate to provide basic information and to counsel patients about proper drug use. Additionally, pharmacists have a tremendous knowledge base about medications. Drug labeling should be a complementary link to physician and pharmacist counseling. However, as demonstrated earlier, health care providers have missed opportunities to counsel patients on the proper use of prescription medications.

Finding number six of the white paper states that "Health care providers are not adequately communicating to patients, either orally or in print, for prescribed medicines. More training is needed to promote best practices for writing prescriptions and counseling patients."

What is needed is an evidence-based approach to drug labeling that includes testing of a new, standard drug label and identification of best practices that are then communicated to physicians and pharmacists. Furthermore, research that incorporates known best practices is needed to determine whether the proposed changes result in improved patient understanding, behaviors, and ultimately health outcomes. Finally, it is crucial that systems of prescribing and dispensing be integrated to provide the best information.

The final finding of the ACP Foundation white paper states that "Research support is necessary to advance the science of drug labeling and identify best practices for patient medication information."

Wolf concluded that variability is most likely a major cause of medication error and that there is evidence to support the conclusion that the way we currently communicate information on prescription medications leads to a variety of problems. The white paper focused on medication container labeling because it may be the most important, most tangible information about use of prescription medications that is actually used by patients. There is an opportunity for improvement through setting evidence-based standards for drug labels. It is also important, Wolf observed, to view drug labeling as a system of patient information that should be integrated into the entire process of prescription, dispensing, and use of prescription medications.

SIMPLIFICATION OF DRUG DOSING TIMES: CAN WE CONFUSE PATIENTS LESS?

Alastair J. J. Wood, M.D., F.A.C.P.
Symphony Capital LLC

Successful drug therapy is dependent upon completing a number of steps accurately. First, a physician must choose the correct drug, make the correct decision about drug dosage, and then correctly write the prescription. A pharmacist must then correctly understand the written prescription, accurately transcribe the prescription to the drug label, and correctly transmit information to the patient. Patients have their own requirements for proper drug use. They must first have access to the medicines, and they must then use the medicines correctly. From the patient's perspective, correct medication use involves both accurately understanding the instructions and knowing how to implement the instructions. Additionally, a patient must be able to integrate taking multiple medicines into a daily schedule and, finally, actually take the medicine.

While there are a number of steps in the process at which interventions to reduce medication errors could be made, the focus of this workshop was on improving medication container labels. To take medicines properly, one needs to know what to take, how many pills to take, and when to take them. What appears simple is actually quite complicated. As discussed earlier, there is tremendous variation in labeling instructions. For example, a written survey examined how the instruction "take one pill a day" is written by prescribers and found that it was written 44 different ways. Even the same prescriber wrote the same instruction in different ways throughout the day.

Similarly, variation at the level of the pharmacist's transcription may arise in a number of ways. A single pharmacist may transcribe the same instruction in different ways at different times, there may be variation across pharmacists in one pharmacy, and there may be variation across different pharmacies (see Figure 2-4). While each of the labels in Figure 2-4 may appear reasonable, they can produce very different outcomes. With Fosomax, for example, if the pill stays in the esophagus it causes irritation, so it is very important after taking Fosomax to remain upright and take fluids so that the pill travels to the stomach and doesn't lodge in the esophagus. Therefore, it is appropriate to place on the label the warning, "do not lie down for at least 30 minutes after taking." However,

Prescription	Examples of Pharmacy "Sig" Interpretations
Lipitor 10 mg tabs Take one tab QD Dispense #30 Indication: for high cholesterol No refills	- "Take one tablet daily." - "Take 1 tablet by mouth for high cholesterol." - "Take one (1) tablet(s) by mouth once a day." - "Take one tablet by mouth every day for high cholesterol."
Fosamax 5 mg tabs Take one tab QD Dispense #30 Indication: osteoporosis prevention Do not lie down for at least 30 minutes	- "Take 1 tablet by mouth daily." - "Take one tablet by mouth every day for osteoporosis prevention. Do not lie down for at least 30 minutes after taking." - "Take 1 tablet every day, 30 minutes before breakfast with a glass of water. Do not lie down." - "Take one tablet every day."
Bactrim DS tabs Take one tab BID Dispense #6 Indication: UTI No refills	- "Take one tablet by mouth twice daily for UTI'" - "Take one tablet by mouth twice daily for urinary tract infection." - "Take 1 tablet by mouth 2 times a day." - "Take 1 tablet twice daily for 3 days."
Ibuprofen 200 mg tabs Take 1-2 tabs TID PRN pain Dispense #30 No refills	- "Take 1 to 2 tablets by mouth as needed for pain." - "Take 1 to 2 tablets by mouth three times daily as needed for pain." - "Take 1 to 2 tablets by mouth as needed for pain. **Not to exceed 4 times a day" - "Take 1 to 2 tablets 3 times a day as needed for pain."

FIGURE 2-4 Transcription of Rx to label imperfect and variable.
SOURCE: ACPF (2007).

two of the four pharmacy labels shown in Figure 2-4 did not provide any instruction at all about remaining upright. And of the two that did, one said simply, "do not lie down." But do not lie down for how long—5 minutes, 30 minutes, 2 hours?

While drug labels vary by pharmacy, an examination of those labels does reveal similarities. For example, the most prominent item on a drug bottle label is the pharmacy name, the second most prominent is the pharmacy telephone number, and the third is the number of refills, Wood stated. Less prominent and less clear are the patient's instructions for use.

As Wolf reported previously, 46 percent of patients misinterpret at least one instruction on a prescription bottle label. Table 2-1 provides examples, taken from a 2007 study by Wolf and colleagues, of how patients misinterpret instructions.

The situation becomes even more complicated with multiple medications. For example, assume a patient must take three medications daily, one medication three times a day (TID), a second medication four times a day (QID), and a third medication twice daily (BID). The schedule for taking such medications might look as shown in Table 2-2.

A universal medication schedule (UMS), where patients take all their medications at breakfast, lunch, dinner, and/or bedtime would simplify drug labeling and make directions more understandable for the patient. If such a schedule were followed for the example illustrated in Table 2-2, rather than taking medication eight times a day, the patient would take medication four times a day at the times shown in Table 2-3. With such a schedule, there would be less likelihood of forgetting to take one's medicines.

TABLE 2-1 Patient Misunderstanding of Medication Instructions

Dosage Instruction	Patient Interpretation
Take one teaspoonful by mouth three times daily	Take three teaspoons daily Take three tablespoons every day Drink it three times a day
Take one tablet by mouth twice daily for 7 days	Take two pills a day Take it for 7 days Take one every day for a week I'd take a pill every day for a week
Take two tablets by mouth twice daily	Take it every 8 hours Take it every day Take one every 12 hours

SOURCE: Wolf et al. (2007).

TABLE 2-2 Schedule for Taking Medications TID, QID, and BID

Time	Med Taken	Time	Med Taken
7:00 a.m.	TID med	4:00 p.m.	
8:00 a.m.	QID med	5:00 p.m.	
9:00 a.m.	BID med	6:00 p.m.	
10:00 a.m.		7:00 p.m.	QID med
11:00 a.m.		8:00 p.m.	
Noon		9:00 p.m.	BID med
1:00 p.m.	QID med	10:00 p.m.	
2:00 p.m.		11:00 p.m.	TID and QID med
3:00 p.m.	TID med		

SOURCE: Wood (2007).

TABLE 2-3 Simplified Medication Schedule for TID, QID, and BID

Time of Day	TID	QID	BID
Breakfast	X	X	X
Lunch	X	X	
Dinner		X	X
Bedtime	X	X	

SOURCE: Wood (2007).

Wood reported that a study by Wolf demonstrated that 77 percent of prescriptions could be easily accommodated by the UMS (personal communication, Michael Wolf, Northwestern University Feinberg School of Medicine, October 2007). Of the 346,000 oral prescriptions examined, the study found the following:

- 51 percent were once a day.
- 19 percent were twice a day.
- 5 percent were three times a day.
- 2 percent were four times a day.

If one included prescriptions for medications that were not timed at all—for example, those with instructions to take as directed or as needed—92 percent of all prescriptions could be accommodated with the proposed UMS.

Audience members asked why not specify time intervals (e.g., "take every 6 hours") or specific times a day (e.g., 8:00 a.m. and 8:00 p.m.) rather than using the UMS. In response, Wolf pointed out that studies have shown that hourly intervals are less well understood by patients than directions to take a medication a certain number of times a day. Furthermore, studies using a medication bottle with a chip in the cap that registers when a patient opens the bottle demonstrate that even with specific timed directions for taking a drug, patients do not follow those instructions.

One question is whether a UMS would improve understanding. In a study of 500 patients in two sites in Chicago and Shreveport, Louisiana, Wolf and colleagues compared patients' understanding of instructions for the standard labels for BID, TID, and QID with the UMS (personal communication, Michael Wolf, Northwestern University Feinberg School of Medicine, October 2007). They found that the UMS produced five times better comprehension than the standard labels with a $p < 0.001$. However, as stated in response to a question from the audience, further studies are needed to test the UMS effect on patient understanding.

The UMS also produces an additional benefit: the ability to move to a standard prescription form that would have a schedule that includes breakfast, lunch, dinner, and bedtime (see Figure 2-5). For each prescription medicine, the prescriber could fill in the number of tablets to be

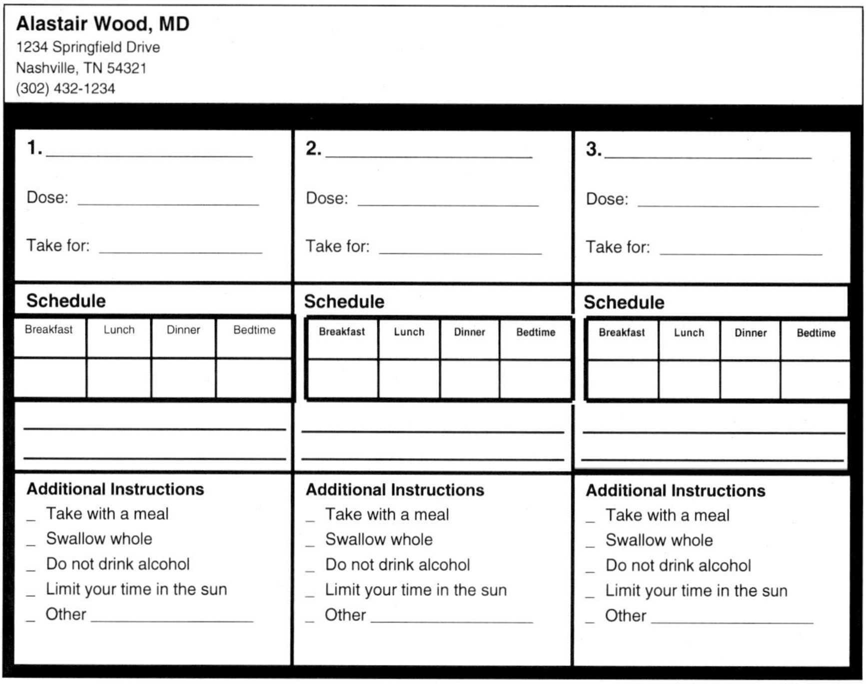

Alastair Wood, MD
1234 Springfield Drive
Nashville, TN 54321
(302) 432-1234

1. ____	2. ____	3. ____
Dose: ____	Dose: ____	Dose: ____
Take for: ____	Take for: ____	Take for: ____
Schedule	**Schedule**	**Schedule**
Breakfast / Lunch / Dinner / Bedtime	Breakfast / Lunch / Dinner / Bedtime	Breakfast / Lunch / Dinner / Bedtime
Additional Instructions	**Additional Instructions**	**Additional Instructions**
_ Take with a meal	_ Take with a meal	_ Take with a meal
_ Swallow whole	_ Swallow whole	_ Swallow whole
_ Do not drink alcohol	_ Do not drink alcohol	_ Do not drink alcohol
_ Limit your time in the sun	_ Limit your time in the sun	_ Limit your time in the sun
_ Other ____	_ Other ____	_ Other ____

FIGURE 2-5 Standard dosing times on prescriptions.
SOURCE: Wood (2007).

taken on the standardized label as well as fill out additional instructions needed.

The standardized prescriptions could then be translated readily onto a standard label on the prescription bottle. Patients, pharmacists, and physicians would all use the same schedule. Variability in prescription writing and transcribing would be reduced substantially, and patients' understanding improved. It is important to note, however, that studies have not been conducted on whether patients' adherence or outcomes would be improved with the UMS.

Additionally, if such a system were adopted, clinical trials of drugs could use UMSs in pivotal clinical trials for FDA approval. Currently, different trials may have different times when drugs are administered as long as the studies adhere to a defined schedule for administration.

A potential objection to use of the UMS is that such a schedule would cause drug concentrations in the body to vary more than would be the case if the patient took the medication at equal intervals—exactly every 8 hours, for example, or exactly every 12 hours. Wood observed that there is greater variation between approved generic drugs and their brand name counterparts than would be the case with administering drugs using the UMS since the FDA requirement for brand/generic equivalence requires only that the 90 percent confidence intervals for peak and average concentrations (AUC) must lie within 80 percent to 125 percent of those of the branded product. Furthermore, concentrations vary enormously among individuals because of biological variability and metabolizing activity. Concentrations can also vary within the same individual because of dietary intake.

In response to questions from the audience, Wood emphasized that the UMS does not remove the need to provide warnings such as can be found on auxiliary labels. It is a system for standardizing the times at which one takes medicine. There are some instances when, for example, taking the medication with certain foods or juices can vastly change the effect of the medication. For those medications, additional instructions should specify which foods to avoid.

Wood concluded that, as data presented in this workshop show, the current situation of drug labeling is unsatisfactory. Prescriptions are unclear. Transcription of a prescription to the label is imperfect. Patients frequently misunderstand the drug label. Finally, variability and complexity of labels are excessive. The potential advantages of the UMS include a simplified dosing schedule with no loss of efficiency, improved patient understanding and patient adherence, reduced errors, reduced variability, and improved therapeutic outcomes.

3

Federal Agency Reaction to Prescription Use Instruction Standardization

CINDY BRACH, M.P.P.

Agency for Healthcare Research and Quality

The evidence is clear that patients do not understand current drug labels, that there are medication adherence problems, and that there are ambulatory medication errors. The presumption is that there is a correlation between understanding and adherence. What is less clear is what should be placed on drug labels to remedy the problems, despite some good best practices from the health literacy research literature as well as specific testing of different labeling approaches.

There is some information about how to improve labels, yet more research is needed to determine what changes to make. Furthermore, there is no strong evidence to demonstrate that changing the label and increasing understanding will lead to better adherence, fewer adverse consequences, or better patient outcomes. More research is needed on these issues. It is also important to address the issue of language barriers in patient understanding of medication information.

The American College of Physicians (ACP) Foundation white paper suggested that a regulatory approach could be used to achieve standardization. There is no good evidence to suggest that regulation is the best approach. However, research about other kinds of medication information shows that voluntary approaches have not been highly successful.

Several questions need to be addressed: What are the mechanisms by which standardization can be achieved? What would the process look like? What are the costs of standardizing? What level of evidence is needed to introduce a best practice? One may be willing to adopt what looks to be an improvement, even without the highest bar of evidence, if the cost is low. However, if there is a high cost, then more evidence is required.

The benefits of standardization have been well presented. The main risk may relate to the energy required to implement a standardized drug label. That is, those efforts might detract from other efforts that are needed to address the problems of low adherence and medication errors.

The Agency for Healthcare Research and Quality (AHRQ) is engaged in a number of activities related to drug labeling and patient understanding. For example, AHRQ has been working with the National Council for Prescription Drug Programs on a program related to standardization in ePrescribing.[1] It is important to examine whether the standardized message the pharmacist receives from the physician is actually a good message to put on the pill label.

AHRQ has also been working on the opportunities for counseling about medications. There are opportunities in inpatient care for discharge education and counseling. A number of projects have been funded in this area, and some of them have developed pictorial graphic pill calendars for patients that display the schedule for their medications. Another project has developed a pill card that is currently being tested. When a patient fills a new prescription at the pharmacy, he or she will receive a pill card with a list of all the medications that have been filled at that pharmacy and instructions for how to take them. The pill card uses various icons such as the sun to indicate morning and the moon to indicate night. The project has also developed a health literacy assessment guide. The guide is used by pharmacies to determine how well they are doing in communicating with their patients and addressing variable health literacy.

AHRQ is also involved in a project called "Questions Are the Answer." Research has shown that patients who leave a provider's office with questions are more likely to have a patient safety event. Thus, a website that aids patients in constructing a list of pertinent questions to ask their doctors has been developed for patients to use before their appointments. The project has also developed a musical public service announcement. And AHRQ is developing a health literacy assessment of patients' experiences, including a question about how easy it was to understand the medication instructions given by the physician.

---

[1]ePrescribing is defined as "the transmission, using electronic media, of prescription or prescription-related information, between a prescriber, dispenser, PBM, or health plan, either directly or through an intermediary, including an ePrescribing network. E-prescribing includes, but is not limited to, two-way transmissions between the point of care and the dispenser" (Federal Register, 2005).

Brach concluded that there will always be some people who do not understand instructions, no matter how carefully the label is written. Therefore, drug labeling needs to be part of an overall strategy to improve medication adherence and reduce medication errors.

NANCY OSTROVE, Ph.D.

Food and Drug Administration

The Food and Drug Administration (FDA) supports evidence-based standardization as a baseline for information accessibility as demonstrated through FDA regulations that require nutrition-facts panels on foods and drug-facts labels for over-the-counter products. Consistently placed information assists the targeted audience in finding information, read the information, and, it is hoped, apply the information. Standardization may be particularly important for populations with limited literacy.

The majority of the findings in the ACP Foundation white paper are well supported by the literature. A major strength of the white paper lies in its proposal for standardization of dosing instructions to the degree to which the implementation of those standards is evidence based. The question is, What specific standard for dosing information will improve understanding and appropriate use of prescription medications, especially for those with lower literacy and health literacy skills? Unfortunately, there is a risk that the desire to rapidly achieve standardization could undermine appropriate research.

For many years, FDA has deferred to state regulations and state boards of pharmacy in determining what information should appear on prescription drug container labels. In fact, there are many who believe that prescription medications are exempted from the Federal Food, Drug and Cosmetic Act requirements for providing adequate directions for use. For the FDA to establish a requirement or set a standard concerning drug labels would be viewed as interfering with the practice of pharmacy. Once a drug is approved for marketing, prescribers are free to prescribe it consistent with their clinical judgment. The FDA does not have the authority to dictate to prescribers how they should write their prescriptions.

Information surrounding the container label (i.e., patient package inserts) is regulated by the FDA. In response to the Institute of Medicine (IOM) report on the future of drug safety (IOM, 2007) and with information obtained from public meetings, the FDA Center for Drug Evaluation and Research is putting together a strategic risk communication plan that will include an examination of all the tools currently used by FDA for communicating drug information. Furthermore, even though consumer medication information sheets are not regulated by the FDA, Congress has mandated that FDA assess the program's success and has defined success as 95 percent of patients in the year 2006 who received new prescriptions also having received useful information with their prescriptions.

FDA has also recently established a Risk Communication Advisory Committee that will provide a forum for discussion of issues and approaches to improving how FDA is communicating with its targeted audiences—both patients and health care providers. The committee will not be addressing specific drug issues or specific device issues but rather will focus on broader issues, such as health literacy and how to appropriately communicate both the risks and benefits of the products FDA regulates from foods through biologics, drugs, and medical devices.

The FDA agrees that standardization is a good idea and that implementation should be evidence based. Implementation could occur through the National Association of Boards of Pharmacy (NABP) and the state boards of pharmacy. The NABP has, for example, a set of model laws that could incorporate standards for prescription container labels. Finally, the FDA does not perceive that existing federal regulations would interfere with implementing standardization.

VIRGINIA TORRISE, Pharm.D.

Department of Veterans Affairs

As a comprehensive health care system, the Department of Veterans Affairs (VA) may face challenges that differ slightly from those encountered in the private sector. The VA serves approximately 5 million veteran patients and dispenses approximately 120 million prescriptions a year. It serves an aging population, the average age of which is approximately 65 years old. Understanding the instructions through the health care process is challenging.

The VA has ePrescribing, it has treatment guidelines, and it will be developing more robust decision support systems. Currently the VA is examining standardization of nomenclature as part of its ePrescribing, a result of an initiative that merged the prescription portion of VA's electronic medical record information system with that of the Department of Defense. Phase II of the merger will examine laboratory information. The VA is also building a personal health record that not only provides information about medications, but will also provide such things as reminders to patients of appointments and upcoming laboratory work. Additionally, if individual patients agree, community providers can include information in the records and patients can list over-the-counter items they purchase.

The VA system integrates the prescribing and filling of prescriptions with an examination of patient understanding and adherence. An important component of proper prescription use is communication from the provider to the pharmacist about the purpose of the prescribed medication. There may also be future opportunities to provide the pharmacist with additional information that will allow him or her to assess, for example, whether a laboratory goal has been met or if there have been risks occurring with certain medications. Pharmacists in the VA work with medical teams, often in clinic settings, where they review the appropriateness of the medication on a medical record, counsel patients, and check to see if patients understand instructions. One approach includes shared appointments, where patients meet with several providers (e.g., physician, nurse, nutritionist, pharmacist) at the same time who communicate with the patient about his or her health and treatment.

The VA shares the commitment to improve health literacy and supports the need for medication label changes but believes such changes should be just one part of a larger approach that must include accessible, verbal communication.

DISCUSSION

An audience member asked if, without considering whether it is the correct thing to do, it would it be possible to write federal legislation or regulations that would mandate standardized drug labeling. Brach stated that the Medicare Prescription Drug, Improvement and Modernization Act of 2003 actually mandates the adoption of standards for interoperability for ePrescribing so that from the prescriber to the pharmacist, there will be a standard. One might say, therefore, that standardization has a legislative basis.

Ostrove responded that it is probably possible, but one then must ask whether it would be the most appropriate approach. Given the historical deferment to the states, the practicality of federal regulation is probably fairly limited. There would most likely be objections about interference with the practice of pharmacy and the practice of medicine.

Panelists were asked, if everyone seems to agree that standardizing the drug label is a good idea, how can this be accomplished without an accompanying policy change? How will these standards be enforced? For example, current evidence shows that despite extremely detailed guidance on the development of FDA medication guides, this guidance is not followed. Should standards be developed and merely circulated with the hope that they will be adopted? Should there be a model practice act developed that is similar to the new California law? While some best practices have been identified, there is no real incentive for their adoption. One can travel through each of the 50 states in the United States and know what a stop sign looks like, but there is no consistency about what a "no food" symbol on a prescription bottle looks like. What will cause the situation to change?

Ostrove responded that these are issues of implementation and raise the overall question of whether the introduction of standards should be a grassroots approach or whether it should be through legislation and regulation. Even if one were to implement regulations, it does not mean that practice will conform, as seen from research that shows mandated medication guides are not distributed. Brach responded that from the perspective of a non-regulatory federal agency, there are options short of regulation, such as working with relevant associations and organizations. If there is sufficient evidence to support standardization, then one could bring relevant groups together to develop an implementation strategy. Such groups might include the Department of Health and Human Services, private-sector partners from relevant associations (e.g., from pharmacy and medicine), and the IOM Roundtable on Health Literacy.

The panel was then asked whether the expanding use of electronic medical records presents any additional regulatory or legislative possibilities or issues. Brach responded that, to her knowledge, there are no prohibitions to such legislation or regulation. Currently there are a number of systems operating. The Department of Health and Human Services is engaged in trying to reach a consensus about interoperability among the many vendors of the systems that do exist, but it is not pursuing regulation in this area. Torrise agreed that there is probably nothing that would prevent such regulation, but there are disincentives.

Panelists were then asked if each would state who should take leadership on moving forward on the issue of drug label standardization. Torrise stated that since the VA is, in effect, its own state board of pharmacy, it can write the necessary policies for its system. Furthermore, the VA will be closely examining the issue of standardization to determine how to move forward in this area. Brach suggested that the implementation issues are beyond the purview of one federal agency and, instead, require the cooperation of all those involved. From the AHRQ perspective, Brach stated, one needs to determine how drug label standardization would be integrated into the overall strategies of improving other pieces of the system, such as patient counseling, since merely standardizing drug labeling would not fix the problems of medication safety and adherence.

Ostrove agreed with Brach and further pointed out that there is as yet no information on the impact of such standardization on patient adherence. Until that is available, the best that can be done is to develop a theoretical marketing plan for the idea. Groups that could be instrumental in moving forward with this include the IOM, working very closely with the pharmacy industry and the NABP.

4

Reaction from the Pharmacy Field to Prescription Use Instruction Standardization

ALAN GOLDHAMMER, Ph.D.

Pharmaceutical Research and Manufacturers of America

For the issues under discussion, the pharmaceutical industry role is primarily limited to packaging pharmaceuticals and moving them into the supply chain, where they are shipped to pharmacies and dispensed. Everything done by the industry is regulated by the Food and Drug Administration (FDA), down to the letters used on the drug label. Unless a pharmaceutical manufacturer is supplying items in unit-of-use packaging (e.g., oral contraceptive pills), the drugs are usually shipped in large bottles that are then repackaged by the pharmacist in smaller containers with medication labels affixed at that point. However, what the industry does in unit-of-use packaging is done effectively and probably addresses a number of the issues under discussion.

Physicians, pharmacists, and patients all have responsibilities in ensuring appropriate medication use. Patients have the responsibility to request information from their physicians and, if they need additional information, from their pharmacists. Furthermore, patients should have a written medication record, that is, a record of all the medicines they are taking. Pharmacists have a responsibility to counsel patients. However, given that pharmacists are frequently overworked, there is insufficient time to provide the kind of counseling needed. What pharmacists can do is dispense consumer medication information leaflets and draw patients' attention to the information. Physicians need to learn to write prescriptions clearly and to ensure that appropriate information is given to patients; ultimately, these are skills that should be included in the medical school curriculum.

Drug labels need to be made much simpler. An important partner in determining how to move forward in this process is the National Association of Boards of Pharmacy.

DARREN K. TOWNZEN, R.Ph., M.B.A.

Director of Pharmacy Systems, Wal-Mart

An expected benefit of standardization is consistency. Clearly there is now great inconsistency across pharmacies. As Wolf stated when describing the 31 different label styles developed in response to state regulations, there is great disparity in minimal requirements. It is to the benefit of a chain such as Wal-Mart that as much information as possible is presented in a consistent manner.

However, there are barriers and limitations to standardization. One barrier is the opportunity costs of standardization. That is, if improvement efforts are focused on standardization, it could result in not implementing other approaches to reducing medication errors that might have a bigger effect on consumer health and well-being. Another concern relates to adopting a standard that requires placing the indication for the medication on the label. Some patients may not wish such information displayed on the label—for example, patients who are being treated for depression or erectile dysfunction. In determining the information that should appear on a label, the patient's perspective should be considered.

There are some advantages to unit-of-use packaging such as the Z-Pak (Zithromax®) developed by Pfizer. For example, regardless of what the physician writes on the prescription or what the pharmacy provides the patient when it dispenses the medication, necessary information is consistently presented on the Z-Pak itself, including what the medication is for and how to take it. The packaging also includes the lot number and expiration date, which would be of great value if a Class I recall was issued.

Wal-Mart is examining the possibility of placing generic medication in a package similar to that of the Z-Pak, always being cognizant of current FDA restrictions, and is working with the generic manufacturers to accomplish this. The approach was tested with Warfarin. Consumers were presented with the medication in what is called consumerized prescription packaging. The responses were very positive.

An examination of the current evidence seems to support standardization of drug labels as a mechanism for increasing patient comprehension. However, increasing comprehension is not the same as increasing adherence. It is likely that even with inventive approaches to increasing patient understanding, many patients will not take their medication as directed. Therefore, a variety of approaches are needed to solve current problems.

GERALD McEVOY, Pharm.D.

American Society of Health-System Pharmacists

As a professional practice association that represents pharmacists, the American Society of Health-System Pharmacists (ASHP) is very supportive of the recommendations of the ACP Foundation white paper and the need for standardization. There is clear evidence documenting problems, and the ASHP believes that medication labeling standards are one part of the solution. While best practices are described here and in the white paper (e.g., simplified statements and formatting issues), evidence to support a particular approach is lacking. Furthermore, the ultimate outcome of suggested changes has not yet been established, either for medication safety or for patient adherence.

The use of regulation as a solution is of great concern. For instance, medication guides are an example of how the FDA has regulated a pharmacy practice issue. These guides have not been a success for many reasons, one of which is the FDA's failure to understand the basic dispensing function. While there are well-established standards for content and format of these guides, many of them have become focused on a single risk without any description of benefit and without incorporating all the standards for content and format. Following a regulatory approach could result in a very long wait for gains to be realized.

The ASHP is involved in many initiatives that address the issues discussed here and in the ACP Foundation white paper. It has an extensive and well-established policy development process with key groups that include the Section on Pharmacy, Informatics, and Technology, the Council of Therapeutics, and a center on patient safety. Key guidelines have been developed for patient education and counseling that include the core recognition that pharmacists have a responsibility to provide counseling, not just to offer it. Furthermore, the ASHP is a publisher of consumer medication information (CMI), is a resource used by the National Library of Medicine's Medline Plus, has a working relationship with Consumer Reports that can be used to educate consumers, and operates the website SafeMedications.com.

Several difficulties must be considered when designing solutions to the problems associated with drug container labeling. One question raised earlier related to the costs estimated for implementing changes. Given the number of systems in place that would be affected, such as legacy (old) computer systems, the costs could be considerable. Furthermore, the evidence required to substantiate a large investment in a particular approach to standardized labels is lacking. Another difficulty is changing long-standing professional practice, both in medicine and pharmacy.

For pharmacists in hospital settings, times for administration of medication are driven by when nurses typically make rounds to distribute medications. In the ambulatory setting this is not the case, which complicates the standardization process. Medication reconciliation,[1] required by the Joint Commission on Accreditation of Healthcare Organizations, is another key issue that will affect attempts at standardization, as will computerized physician order entry (CPOE) systems. Each CPOE vendor can independently develop the dosage instructions available through the CPOE. For standardization to work in both the hospital and the ambulatory settings, there must be some effort to bring concordance to these systems.

Currently, the National Council for Prescription Drug Programs (NCPDP) is focusing on standards for communication between the prescriber and the pharmacist. It also has a strong international influence. However, the Department of Veterans Affairs principally uses standards from HL7.[2] There are efforts under way to ensure the standards are in agreement, which is very important, but one must also take into account issues related to how international recommendations would relate to the U.S. model of health care. Finally, one must address issues surrounding the use of legacy systems as well as physician and pharmacist behaviors.

Medication safety is a professional practice issue. It involves the professions of pharmacy and medicine as well as other health care providers involved in counseling patients about safe and effective medication use. The ASHP does not believe that regulation, at least as an initial approach, is the appropriate avenue to follow. Rather, the focus should be on developing best practices that are evidence based and have a broad base of stakeholder input.

---

[1]Reconciliation is the process of comparing what medication the patient is taking at the time of admission or entry to a new setting or level of care with what the organization is providing (admission or new medication orders) in order to avoid errors such as conflicts or unintentional omissions (AAP, 2005).

[2]Health Level 7 (HL7) refers both to an organization involved in setting international health care standards and to some of the specific standards it has developed. HL7 are "ANSI-accredited standards for electronically defining clinical and administrative data in the healthcare industry. HL7 is one of several Standards Developing Organizations in healthcare. The '7' comes from application layer 7 in the OSI model, which is the highest level where programs talk to each other" (*PC Magazine,* 2007).

The ASHP does support a broadly based stakeholder process for investigating the problems and the best means for establishing needed standards. Organizations that should participate in this process include the National Association of Boards of Pharmacy (NABP), the NCPDP, HL7, the Joint Commission, the United States Pharmacopeia (USP), and, given the emergence of ePrescribing models and other informatics initiatives, the American Medical Informatics Association (AMIA).

WILLIAM ELLIS, R.Ph., M.S.
American Pharmacists Association Foundation

The IOM Roundtable on Health Literacy and the ACP Foundation are to be commended for convening this group and undertaking the task of examining problems and solutions for the issues surrounding medication container labeling. There is certainly evidence to support standardization of medication labeling. The time is right in health care, and more specifically in pharmacy practice, to begin discussing needed changes, since there is a great deal of discussion occurring about changing the basic model of pharmacy practice and moving to a more patient-centered approach.

Medications are among our most powerful tools in the fight against disease. Yet medications are frequently viewed as simple commodities. When that occurs, one begins to lose the ability to differentiate among them. Patients assume all medications have been approved by the FDA and that they are therefore safe and effective. Furthermore, patients often believe that over-the-counter medications cannot cause harm. It is important that pharmacists and physicians communicate that medications, whether over-the-counter products or prescription medications, must be used respectfully.

While it is important from a quality improvement perspective to address prescription labeling, it is also important not to lose sight of the larger picture in which health care is delivered, a picture that includes interactions between patients, pharmacists, physicians, and other health care providers. Labeling must be examined against this broader system, and an important tool in this examination is practice-based research.

The American Pharmacist Association (APhA) Foundation conducts practice-based research related to improving outcomes in chronic disease through a variety of initiatives such as the Diabetes Ten City Challenge,[3]

---

[3]The Diabetes Ten City Challenge is a program for use by employers and communities to address diabetes and reduce health care costs through implementation of the APhA Foundation's Patient Self-Management Program. Using incentives, employer groups in 10 communities, with the help of pharmacist coaches, physicians, and community health resources, encourage people to manage their diabetes (APhA, 2007).

which is a highly collaborative effort involving teams of physicians, pharmacists, nurses, diabetes educators, and patients. Such research will help identify best practices, which are to be preferred over a regulatory approach.

While regulation is not favored as the primary approach to solve drug labeling problems, there may be some role for regulation. For example, the NABP plays an important role in developing model regulations for review and use by the 50 state boards of pharmacy. In moving forward to address the kinds of issues raised here, thought could be given to a national collaboration that would examine how to implement some of the best practices we know exist. There are numerous stakeholders that should participate in such an effort, many of whom have already been identified. Although it is important to hold discussions of how to proceed, action is also necessary.

DISCUSSION

One participant asked, since those on the panel appear to favor moving forward with standardization and the recommendations in the ACP Foundation white paper, who should lead that effort? Goldhammer responded that the leader should come from the field of pharmacy. Townzen suggested that the NCPDP would be an appropriate leader. That organization has been identified by the Consolidated Health Initiative as an appropriate group for establishing standards. Furthermore, the NCPDP has devised a standardized prescription card to address some of the variation in state requirements. McEvoy agreed that the NCPDP is a key participant and reiterated what he stated during his presentation, that is, that the other groups that should be involved include the AMIA, USP, the Joint Commission, HL7, and the IOM. McEvoy also suggested that one might wish to have a neutral convener for this effort, perhaps a new consortium of groups. Ellis responded that medicine and pharmacy practitioner organizations should begin the process but that other stakeholders should be involved.

Panelists were asked whether there are business or competitive issues (other than costs of implementation) to consider that might create barriers to implementation if efforts to standardize labels resulted in minimizing pharmacy logos. Ellis and Townzen agreed that the effect of minimizing the pharmacy logo is probably minimal and should not impede implementation.

Another questioner asked whether clinical trials could be designed around a standard medication administration schedule and, if so, whether pharmaceutical manufacturers could take the lead on that restructuring. Goldhammer responded that it seems possible to structure clinical trials to include standardized administration and that it would be appropriate for the pharmaceutical industry to investigate this.

5

Other Stakeholder Reaction to Prescription Use Instruction Standardization: Physicians and Patients

WILLIAM DOLAN, M.D.

American Medical Association

The Institute of Medicine Roundtable on Health Literacy and the American College of Physicians (ACP) Foundation are to be commended for their work in the area of standardizing drug labels. There is a crisis. One in seven people in the United States is without health insurance, but about one in three (90 million people) cannot read their prescription labels and are uninformed about the treatment they are receiving. While there may be disagreements with some portions of the ACP Foundation white paper, the American Medical Association (AMA) supports the exploration of a standard medication label format.

There are many causes of the problems that face us, including, for example, the poor reading skills of many American citizens. However, addressing the labeling problems is a proper place to begin our efforts to improve patient understanding. Drug labeling changes might be implemented on a state-by-state basis, as is occurring with attempts to provide health insurance to the uninsured. States have the capacity to make changes. Chain stores such as Wal-Mart and Target are other places to begin change efforts.

Changing the format in which physicians write prescriptions is probably not the best approach. Using Latin to inform the pharmacist has worked well. Furthermore, states have their own requirements. New York, for instance, has recently developed a tamper-proof prescription pad that every physician is required to use. Mandating a uniform prescription pad across all states would require legislation. Congress has been considering legislation that would require all Medicaid prescriptions be tamper proof, but it is currently on hold because of numerous problems.

Widespread use of electronic medical records may lead to prescription format changes. However, only 10 percent of physicians currently have electronic medical records. They are very costly—about $30,000 to $50,000 per physician per setup, with a $1,000 monthly maintenance fee. Furthermore, because there are between 100 and 300 providers of the software for electronic medical records, interoperability is a problem.

Improving patient understanding requires better physician counseling. The AMA has a large literacy program with workbooks for clinicians and others, as well as patient handouts. There are also movies about health literacy available on the AMA website.

The AMA supports efforts aimed at improving patient understanding and will work with others to accomplish this. In response to a question from the audience, Dolan agreed that there should be a convening organization—perhaps the National Patient Safety Foundation, the IOM, or the AMA—to bring together interested stakeholders. There should also be broad collaboration of all stakeholders in the effort.

ALBERT WU, M.D., M.P.H.

Bloomberg School of Public Health, Johns Hopkins University

There is enough evidence available to show that something must be done to address problems with patient understanding and use of medications. The question is, What should be done? To answer this question, evidence tables are needed that delineate the level of evidence available for each of the recommendations made in the white paper and for the specific proposal for standardization. A research agenda to evaluate the effectiveness of different strategies is needed as well.

There are several challenges that will be encountered as one moves forward with standardizing medication container labels. One of the challenges of standardization is that there must be room for exceptions. All guidelines are applicable in 80 percent or 90 percent of the cases, but they must be written to allow room for improvisation because there are always nonstandard orders that need to be written. Another challenge is the writing of prescriptions. Handwriting as a method for getting prescriptions into the medication system is one of the root causes of variability and should be eliminated. It is important to take action before ePrescribing is in widespread use so that the systems will be interoperable. A third challenge is that the business case for standardization has not been made. What will standardization cost? Yet another challenge is that there is not, at present, sufficient outrage about the problems of the current system of medication drug labeling. How many people really think there is a problem in prescription writing and dispensing? The issues need to be well publicized.

There is also tension between innovation and standardization. There is an opportunity for research given the innovations that organizations such as Pfizer, Target, Wal-Mart, and the Department of Veterans Affairs are undertaking in this area. At the same time there is the proposal for standardization put forth by Wood at this conference and the approach being taken in California. Studies are needed to compare the effectiveness of various approaches, using logic models to examine outcomes. Such outcomes include understanding, adherence, medication errors, and injuries. However, it is important to remember that when something new is implemented, it is very likely that performance will become slightly worse before improvements are made. As efforts are evaluated, this must be kept in mind.

Policy change is needed. There are local policy changes in systems that cover millions of people (e.g., California, Veterans Affairs, Wal-Mart). However, more evidence is needed before national policy can be developed. National policy is necessary to compel practice change.

To lead this effort a convener is needed. The IOM, by virtue of having assembled such an impressive group of people at this conference, has begun the process. Perhaps the National Quality Forum could play a major role. Constituents from across the medication use spectrum are needed in the effort, not just those from health literacy, but from a much broader base.

WILLIAM BULLMAN, M.A.M.

National Council on Patient Information and Education

The expertise that has been brought to bear on the production of the white paper and the organization of this conference is tremendous. The ACP Foundation and the IOM Roundtable on Health Literacy are to be commended. The white paper is comprehensive. The presentation regarding the universal medication schedule was fascinating.

What, then, are the next steps needed? The call for regulation may be premature. The experience of the National Council on Patient Information and Education (NCPIE) might be brought to bear in an examination of this issue. The NCPIE has been involved in attempting to stimulate quality improvements in written drug information, both in the clinical content and the design layout and readability of the consumer medical information sheets. Furthermore, it has convened groups to discuss with the FDA issues related to the medication guide and the concept of the electronic medication guide. Efforts in this area call into question the idea that regulation is a panacea, and caution is urged in pursuing the regulatory avenue.

The NCPIE was formed in 1982 with a mission to stimulate and improve communication of information on appropriate medicine use. The operating philosophy is that oral counseling, supported by appropriately designed written information as adjunctive information, is the way to achieve a more informed patient or caregiver.

An examination of data from about 1992 to 2004 will show that consumers are not routinely receiving information about instructions for use, precautions and warnings, side effects, and refills. Only about 60 percent to 64 percent of patients report receiving information in the physician's office—primarily about refills and side effects—and the figures are even lower for pharmacies. At the same time, patients have failed to ask for information. Increasing these percentages requires behavioral change, an extremely difficult challenge.

We are not without tools. The AMA has guidelines for counseling patients in the ambulatory care setting. There are counseling guidelines for pharmacy and nursing guidelines about appropriate medication communication. These have not, however, undergone any kind of rigorous research program to determine if they are effective or to learn how to make them better.

Addressing the issue of drug label standardization, the United States Pharmacopeia might be a very good place to move this initiative forward. It has a committee on safe medication use and is involved with the National Coordinating Council for Medication Error Reporting and Prevention (NCC MERP). Furthermore, it has a multidisciplinary membership that includes federal agencies.

LINDA WEISS, Ph.D.

New York Academy of Medicine

The ACP Foundation white paper advocates standardization of prescription drug container labels. Standardization would also facilitate translation of instructions into other languages. As Wood reported, the instruction "take 1 pill a day," was written in 44 different ways. Translating the instruction once, from a standard format, is reasonable; expecting pharmacists to provide 44 translations is likely to cause a number of problems.

The white paper concluded that improvements are also needed in other sources of consumer medication information. These improvements should include, for example, standardized translation of medication labels and other information provided during the pharmacy's medication counseling.

The New York Academy of Medicine has been working in the area of translated medication information for patients who do not speak English well. Results of a study on access to translated medication labels were used by the Academy to develop a continuing education curriculum for pharmacists as well as other interventions for use in New York City. Work is being undertaken collaboratively with physicians, nurses, pharmacists, health educators, and immigrant advocates.

New York City is home to 2.9 million foreign-born people. Almost half of New York City residents speak a language at home other than English. More than one in four adults say they do not speak English well, and about half of those are in homes where no one speaks English well.

Increasingly, limited English proficiency is a national issue. Between 1990 and 2000, 45 states saw growth in their immigrant populations, some by 300 percent or 400 percent. In the country as a whole, some 21 million people say they are limited English proficient, a growth rate of 50 percent over the past decade. Research suggests that patients who do not speak English well have poor knowledge of medication and dosing instructions as well as significantly greater problems with medication adherence and that providing oral and written medication information in their language is linked to improved health outcomes.

The New York Academy of Medicine conducted a random sample telephone survey of 200 pharmacies. The survey found that 88 percent reported that they served patients daily who did not speak English well. Eighty percent stated that they could translate labels into at least one language. But of those with daily limited English proficiency patients, fewer than 40 percent translated daily, while almost 25 percent never translated. Some 88.5 percent of the 200 pharmacies employed bilingual staff, but less than half of these staff were pharmacists or pharmacy interns. It was found that in many of these pharmacies, counseling was being provided by store cashiers or by another customer in the store.

The study and follow-up discussions identified a number of factors associated with limited access to the use of translated medication information. One factor is capacity. Dispensing software may not have translation capacity or the capacity to translate into needed languages. A related factor is concern about the accuracy and reliability of translations that are provided. Some systems are better than others. Pharmacists reported that they have often identified errors in their English labels and therefore expect that such errors also exist in the translations. Pharmacists who do not speak the language are concerned that the instructions and other information might not be correct.

Another concern is that many software systems can print in one language only. If the label is translated, then it is entirely in the translated language and may not comply with regulations. For pharmacists who cannot read the translated label, there is again concern that the information on the translation might not be correct. Pharmacists were also concerned about the time and the cost of providing translated written materials as well as translated telephone services. A number of pharmacies had such telephone services, but they were not used.

For those who need a translated label, it appears that the mechanics of translation would be facilitated by standardization. Furthermore, to the extent that research will be conducted on label standardization, it makes sense that such research also examine translation of labels. Whatever format is ultimately chosen, provision should be made for translation of that format. Furthermore, there should be a broad collaborative effort involving all the different professions as well as the patient perspective in moving forward with the idea of standardization.

MARA YOUDELMAN, J.D., L.L.M.

National Health Law Program

Of the more than 21 million people in the United States who are limited English proficient (LEP), slightly over 2 million are individuals over age 65. Given what we know about problems in understanding medication instructions among people over 65 who are proficient in English, it is certain that the problems must be worse for those people over 65 who are LEP.

One study conducted in hospitals in the Boston area showed that 27 percent of patients who needed but did not have interpreters left the hospital not knowing how to take their prescription drugs. For those who either did not need an interpreter or for whom interpretations were supplied, only 2 percent did not understand how to take their medications. While the problem for LEP patients cannot be eliminated simply by modifying the medication labels, changing the labels will help significantly.

In addition to the problems that pharmacists face, clinicians also are struggling with how to meet the needs of their LEP patients. The National Health Law Program (NHLP) has surveyed this issue. One such survey conducted with the American Hospital Association found that 81 percent of hospitals are treating LEP individuals at least monthly. Sixty-three percent of these hospitals are seeing LEP patients daily or weekly. The NHLP also conducted a survey with the American College of Physicians that found that about 65 percent of all internists have active patients with LEP and that 81 percent of these physicians are treating LEP patients monthly. Therefore, when we are discussing the issues of understanding and compliance with prescription drug instructions, we must examine not only what happens in pharmacies, but also in the broader medical system.

Legally, standardization would be of great assistance because any clinician who accepts federal funds in the United States is subject to Title VI of the Civil Rights Act of 1964, which states that one cannot discriminate on the basis of national origin. The Supreme Court and the federal agencies have said that language can be a proxy for national origin. Therefore, clinicians treating Medicare, Medicaid, and state children's health insurance program patients have an affirmative expectation to provide language services to meet the needs of their LEP patients.

Having a standard medication label in place eases the ability to translate these labels and therefore will be of great assistance to clinicians and pharmacists in meeting their existing obligations under Title VI. There is nothing in the federal laws that prohibits translation; rather there appears to be a more permissive approach that allows inclusion of other languages in a prescription label.

Some states, such as New York, have provided affirmative support for translation. One of the state pharmacy laws in New York talks about misbranded drugs and says that any word, statement, or other information required to appear on the label must be in terms likely to be read and understood by the ordinary individual. In New York City, as is the case in more and more cities across the country, an ordinary individual would very likely include an LEP individual. Therefore, pharmacists might not be in compliance with state law or might be found to have misbranded a drug if they are not providing the translation.

There is significant support in existing law at both the federal civil rights level and in some states to encourage standardization to ease the way for compliance with these laws. Standardization is essential to ensuring that LEP individuals have the access to the health care system that is guaranteed under federal law. Furthermore, with standardization there would be only one way to write "take one pill a day," and that phrase could be translated by one software company or every software company into the top languages needed, thus easing the burden on pharmacies and pharmacists for multiple translations.

Moving forward with standardization should be a collaborative effort, but who leads that effort depends on which organizations have the relevant expertise, clout, commitment, and interest to bring all the stakeholders together.

DISCUSSION

One audience member stated that an evidence-based standardized format for writing prescriptions would make the job of the physician much easier. With such a standardized form, even if it were translated into another language, the prescriber would know exactly where and how to fill in the instructions for use. Therefore, moving forward with testing of a standardized prescription format appears to be a very good idea.

Another participant raised concerns about samples. In many cases, particularly with vulnerable populations who cannot afford medications and who are seen in community health centers and other settings, physicians often give samples and provide instructions for their use. Providing such samples may be of great concern, particularly when they are given to patients with low levels of literacy or language barriers. Wu responded that the IOM report on preventing medication errors (2007) was quite critical about the use of samples because samples provide many opportunities for bypassing safety checks that otherwise exist. However, if such samples were dispensed in unit-of-use packages, this might be an opportunity to provide more information in an attractive package and might offset some of the potential risks caused by the relatively unfettered distribution of samples. Bullman stated that the NCC MERP is examining the use of samples. Dolan emphasized the need for counseling and education of patients about proper medication use.

6

Other Stakeholder Reaction to Prescription Use Instruction Standardization: Educators of Pharmacists and Physicians

MARY ANN F. KIRKPATRICK, Ph.D.

American Association of Colleges of Pharmacy

Schools of pharmacy are very aware of the need for improvements in prescription medication labeling and counseling to improve health literacy and patient safety. This need is well documented in the literature. There are also additional incentives to include such material in the curriculum. First, the Accreditation Council for Pharmacy Education has established new guidelines that emphasize cultural competence and health literacy. Second, the Joint Commission of Pharmacy Practitioners vision statement says that the foundations of pharmacy practice include optimizing medication therapy via patient-centered practices.

In 2006 the entire interim meeting of the American Association of Colleges of Pharmacy (AACP) focused on cultural competence, closing gaps, and expanding access. Furthermore, there has been a call from the organization for examples of best practices in serving the underserved as well as a call for curricula frameworks for addressing special needs of the underserved. The association also provides online resources that are directly linked with its web page, and the annual meetings have both podium and poster sessions directed to this topic.

Pharmacy students learn the mechanics of labeling in dispensing labs. In the law courses they learn about the legal requirements. In management courses they learn how to select systems, including software systems, that are used for dispensing. Communication courses explain how to augment information on instructions for use of medications, and communication training is enhanced during the introductory pharmacy practice experience as well as in other courses. One of the most popular courses is Spanish for health care providers. The demand for this elective has been so high that professors are brought from the academic campus to the medical campus to teach the courses on-site.

A popular course on the psychosocial aspects of disease includes a description of the effect of health literacy on services received. During service learning experiences students learn about overcoming barriers to access. Internships expose on-the-job students to the unique needs of their patients. There are also national competitions, such as the one on patient counseling sponsored by the American Pharmacists Association, that expose students to these issues.

With all the emphasis on communication and serving the under-served, why do problems with labeling and instructions still exist? What are the barriers to change? State boards of pharmacy regulate the information that must appear on the medication label and, as described earlier, this results in variation in labels. Some state boards of pharmacy do not require the capability of producing labels written in Spanish. Furthermore, how can one determine if the patient needs a label in another language? Does a pharmacist just look at the name and make an assumption? Does he or she wait until the patient comes in to discover if another language is needed? Another barrier relates to the small number of pharmacists who are bilingual or multilingual. Furthermore, there is reluctance to make major label changes.

However, changes are under way. Target, for example, is trying to address some of the problems with its prescription label. The name of the medication is in a large font. Directions are in a large font at the top of the label where they can be seen.

There are also increased dispensing software options. One software company provided a list of 524 different fields for which the pharmacist could suggest medication label changes. Font size on all of those fields can be adjusted for specific patients and also for routine labels. This particular software can print labels in English, Spanish, or French. However, as mentioned previously, the entire label is in one language, and pharmacists who do not speak the language printed on the label are concerned about its accuracy. Auxiliary labels can be printed with or without the icons.

The AACP and other pharmacy organizations are developing data that will help address the problems we have been discussing today. These data will also help in the proper training of students. In responding to a question from the floor, Kirkpatrick stated that pharmacy students are taught how to interpret the physicians' dosage instructions or "sig." However, what is printed on the label is what the pharmacy's software system prints out. Pharmacy students are being prepared to address labeling concerns. Software is being developed that can be manipulated to help address some of the labeling problems. Selected companies are trying to reengineer those labels to come up with new and better approaches.

As a next step, academics need to continue to work with state boards of pharmacy and other stakeholders to address these issues. By law, certain things must be taught to pharmacy students, but best practices must also be taught, and one must be alert to identify these best practices. In response to a question from the floor, Kirkpatrick said that the United States Pharmacopeia could play a major leadership role in the issues of medication labeling.

MERRILL EGORIN, M.D.

University of Pittsburgh School of Medicine

The Association of American Medical Colleges (AAMC) recognizes the problems confronting safe and effective use of medications. Prescribing medications is one of the activities that distinguishes a physician from other health care professionals. It is a privilege that carries with it serious responsibilities to patients, society, and the profession. For these reasons it is important that medical students understand what is involved in good prescribing practices. Additionally, too few physicians possess fundamental understanding of and training in pharmacotherapy and rational prescribing.

It is striking that physicians rarely see their patients' pill bottles and so they are unlikely to have any idea what is written on them. For some patients cost may be a barrier, so it is important to train medical students to call the pharmacy to determine what a prescription will cost.

There have been increasing expressions of concern from physicians in the pharmaceutical industry, from pharmacology faculty, and from residency program directors that medical students are not receiving sufficient education about the process of drug discovery, development, and regulation as well as the knowledge and skills involved in safely prescribing these medications. A group including representatives from the pharmaceutical industry and from U.S. and Canadian medical schools convened to consider this issue for a Medical Schools Objective Project Report.[1] The group considered several questions: What should medical students learn in order to become knowledgeable, safe, and effective prescribers of medicine? What is the ideal educational environment for learning about

---

[1]The Medical Schools Objective Project Reports are sent to all medical schools. They are not binding, but they are suggestions for improvement.

the optimal prescribing of medication? What kind of educational experiences would allow students to achieve those learning objectives? The framework in which this discussion took place was the six core principles recommended by the Accreditation Council for Graduate Medical Education: medical knowledge, patient care, interpersonal communication skills, professionalism, practice-based learning and improvement, and systems-based practice.

A number of suggestions were made, including the need for multidisciplinary involvement, particularly when students and house officers make rounds. It was pointed out that a number of medical schools do not have pharmacy schools associated with them, which is a barrier. Another barrier is the dwindling number of clinical pharmacology divisions.

In response to a question from the floor, Egorin stated that the AAMC is willing to play a leadership role in issues of drug labeling and counseling.

DISCUSSION

Sandra Guckian, from the National Association of Chain Drug Stores, said that the association had been working closely with the American Pharmacists Association to develop educational materials and templates for community pharmacists, both for chain pharmacists and independents. These materials could be used by ambulatory care centers as well. Much effort has focused on medication management and the role of the community pharmacist, particularly with patient populations that suffer from multiple chronic conditions and take multiple medications.

One of the core components of the concept of medication therapy management is the personal medication record, which includes more than the prescription label. Information can be inserted for the patient such as when to take medication and reminders to match a patient's drug regimen to his or her particular lifestyle. The pharmacy can play a key role in developing and maintaining this record.

7

What Would It Take to Move Toward Prescription Use Instruction Standardization?

ROGER WILLIAMS, M.D.

United States Pharmacopeia

The United States Pharmacopeia (USP) is a standard-setting body. There are about 500 standard-setting bodies in the United States. Three hundred or so are accredited by the American National Standard Institute (ANSI), which is a professional association that watches over all the U.S. standard-setting bodies. At the global level there is the International Standards Organization (ISO) in Geneva, Switzerland.

Standards can be either documentary or physical. The USP sells physical reference materials, as does the National Institute of Standards in Technology (NIST). Documentary standards include such things as best practices, guidelines, guidance, regulations, and laws. From this perspective, the patient package insert is a standard.

Standards can be voluntary or mandatory. Additionally, there are different kinds of standard-setting bodies. For example, there are voluntary consensus standard-setting bodies where individuals affected by the standards participate in developing them. Government is a very strong standard-setting body, but that is a different model.

The USP is a convention of about 450 associations, and it is a practitioner-based body. There are about 40 pharmacopeias worldwide, but the only one of them that is nongovernmental is the USP. The USP was started in 1820 by practitioners who desired good standards and good names for the medicines they used.

Good pharmaceutical care involves a long process that begins with drug discovery at one end of the process and moves through many steps until it ends with the patient properly using the drug. In considering how to improve patient outcomes, one can look at any of the component steps in this process, but standardizing prescription medication labels is an issue that deserves consideration and that would have a major impact.

Williams stated that the United States had a gross domestic product of more than $13 trillion in 2006 (Geographic.org, 2007). U.S. health care expenditures are expected to exceed $4 trillion by 2016 (AAOS, 2007). As of 2005, the annual expenditure on prescription drugs alone was more than $200 billion (KFF, 2007), and it is likely the drug bill will move much higher. About half the total value of drugs sold worldwide are sold in the United States, and of those, generics account for about 10 percent of the total cost. Generics are approaching 60 percent of all prescriptions, and it is likely that percentage will increase. Given the value of the prescription drug market, even minor improvements could have a large effect in terms of dollar value.

The Hazard Analysis and Critical Control Points is a food safety system used by the Food and Drug Administration (FDA). One could use a similar approach to examine the process whereby medicine moves from the practitioner's office to the patient's home and to determine where the greatest improvement might be achieved. Another way to think about this is using the Situation Target Proposal. The specific proposal offered here is to use one of USP's expert committees, perhaps the Safe Medication and Use Committee, to start working on a format standard for the prescription bottle label. USP is willing to invite representatives of the Institute of Medicine Roundtable on Health Literacy and the American College of Physicians (ACP) Foundation to its next meeting to discuss possibilities.

There has clearly been tremendous progress on standardizing the label, including examples from Pfizer and some of the major chain drug stores. The USP has well-evolved procedures and processes for how a standard-setting activity should proceed. There is a public notice or comment called Pharmacopeial Forum. All stakeholders could participate in this activity in one way or another. One might use the National Coordinating Council for Medication Errors Reporting and Prevention as a staging area to talk about the various issues related to standardization. It should be possible to come forth with a reasonable, voluntary standard in a fairly short amount of time.

It is important to emphasize that the USP is not an enforcing body. It would be up to other bodies—for example, the FDA or state boards of pharmacy—to adopt the standard if they wished to do so. A standard does not have much meaning unless there is also a conformity-assessment activity for the standard. This is something that the USP could offer. At a minimum, the USP would like to participate in the effort. If medication care can be improved, there is the potential to save a great deal of money—for example, by reducing hospitalizations due to improper use of medications.

DARREN K. TOWNZEN, R.Ph., M.B.A.

National Council for Prescription Drug Programs

Why is a standardized label needed? Clearly, one reason is to increase patient understanding. Another reason is because of the inconsistency across states in the information on the prescription drug label. Beyond the label itself are the problematic auxiliary labels. While they serve a purpose, they are difficult to read and understand.

There was discussion earlier about the pharmacist interpreting the prescription. Rarely is it the case that the pharmacist enters that information into the system. Usually it is a technician, although the pharmacist makes sure the printed label is correct. It seems it would be efficient to have a standardized prescription pad as well as a standardized label. Standardization through ePrescribing is preferable. However, if prescriptions are written on paper, a standardized prescription format could increase the level of understanding and reduce errors.

SUSAN JOHNSON, Pharm.D., Ph.D.

Food and Drug Administration

Drug facts labeling for over-the-counter (OTC) products was developed largely because the printing on the products was ghastly. The labeling had become illegible, and there was no standardization in formatting, presentation, or order of idea. Patients were unable to read the labels. While a great improvement over the previous condition, drug facts labeling does have its limitations as a model to use for standardizing prescription drug labels. For instance, the instruction language did not change, so instructions still read "take one every six to eight hours as needed." Perhaps what California develops will prove a more useful model.

An issue of importance is the attitude of the patient toward the medication. There is the perception that OTC medications cannot cause harm. Patients also often believe that if the physician prescribed the medication, it is safe. People lose sight of the risks. This is of particular concern with specific drugs that have narrow therapeutic windows or with specific populations. For example, medication misuse in infant populations can lead to very serious outcomes. An OTC label states that for children under

2 years, the product should be used at the discretion of the physician. Infants should not be dosed by parents or other health care practitioners. However, that is what is occurring, and there are medication errors made because of such things as the dropper used or the markings on the dropper or dosage cup. All of these concerns are outside the realm of the prescription instruction or other label component. They are beyond the control of the dispensing process. However, they are major factors in how a patient actually uses the medication.

Some have suggested that the FDA has placed limitations on the way in which drug labels can be changed or improved. In reality, the FDA has no interest in limiting innovations. Some of the newest moves from a prescription to an OTC drug are good examples of ways in which manufacturers have created innovations to provide patients with extensive consumer information and extensive packaging to increase comprehension. Such innovations would be welcome in the prescription realm as well.

The people attending this conference have the ideas that can move standardization forward. Looking at high-impact changes, as suggested by Williams, is a good place to start for introducing standards, particularly if one is going to propose federal regulation. As FDA lawyers say, show me the proof this works, show me the proof it does not have a down side, show me that people will not object to it, and show me that it does not make things worse. Such things have high impact and are the things that would most quickly and easily become federal standards.

VANESSA CAJINA, M.P.A.

Latino Coalition for a Healthy California

The need to standardize prescription drug labels has been well outlined. On October 11, 2007, California became the first state in the United States to pass legislation adopting standardized prescription drug labeling. The Latino Coalition for a Healthy California (LCHC) has been active in the passage of this legislation, particularly since 20 percent of those living in California speak some language other than English at home. These individuals have poor health outcomes and great health disparities, partially due to an inability to understand the content on prescription drug labels.

LCHC paired with two senior citizen advocacy organizations, the Senior Action Network and the Grey Panthers of California, to investigate the need for standardizing prescription drug labels. Given that research results indicated that the standardized label was more comprehensible, LCHC and its partners worked for passage of legislation to create such a standard label. There are certainly a number of points at which communication about medication can and should occur, including when physicians and pharmacists counsel patients. Labeling, however, is the primary method of communication with a patient and the easiest to legislate.

Legislation was introduced about a year ago by State Senator Ellen Corbett. Initially, many pharmacy associations expressed concern. The LCHC and its partners worked with the associations and with the California State Board of Pharmacy, and in the end these organizations became supporters of the bill, working with the LCHC and its partners to rewrite language and develop a solution to standardizing prescription drug labels.

The new law requires the California Board of Pharmacy to adopt a standardized prescription label by January 1, 2011. The label must take into account input from public meetings and medical literacy research regarding comprehension of labels. The label must have improved directions for use and improved font types and sizes. It must also have patient-centered information placement. The needs of LEP patients, the needs of senior citizens, and technology requirements necessary to implement the standards must be considered. The LCHC and its partners will begin holding stakeholder meetings in January 2008 to develop recommendations for the Board of Pharmacy.

DISCUSSION

One participant stated that it is important to support more research on standardization and that the universal medication system proposed by Wood should be part of any such study. In response, Williams stated that if one waits for all the evidence one wants, there will never be a standard. There are things that can be done now. Another participant suggested that now is a good time to conduct research and evaluation in California, given passage of the law requiring development of a standard drug label.

One audience member asked whether there was a list of preferred ways to provide medication instructions. In response, it was stated that the USP does have available pictograms, allied with standard wording, that were developed several years ago. These have been broadly accepted, even internationally. Currently, the USP is entering into a research agreement with the International Pharmaceutical Federation to test these pictograms as well as some others that have been developed outside the country. As one thinks about changing auxiliary labels, one might consider how to integrate pictograms for better understanding by the patient.

8

Closing Remarks

RUTH PARKER, M.D.

Emory University School of Medicine

Picking up a pill bottle and following the instructions for use is a patient-centered activity. It is what patients need to do; it is at the intersection of understanding and adherence. Being patient centered is one of the hallmarks of quality.

However, medication labels are complex. The whole area of providing drug information is complex. Health literacy is a cross-cutting issue in drug labeling that can impact quality. Health literacy research can help figure out what needs to be done to change the labels so that the patients understand medication instructions. It would be great to see a time when patients look at their pill bottles, look at the instructions on those bottles, understand what they are supposed to do, and safely and effectively take their medications.

Simplifying drug labels sounds like a simple thing, but the devil is in the details. This workshop has discussed the layers of complexity in solving the problems of poor patient understanding of medication instructions, but if one thinks about it, it would be pretty hard to do a worse job than we are doing today. Each person who spoke today acknowledged that there is a problem in drug labeling. Most agreed that standardization would be an improvement. As for regulation, there were some who favored that approach and others who did not.

Courageous leadership is needed to solve the problem. Putting the patient at the center and figuring out what is best for the patient should be the unifying theme. The problems of drug labeling and patient understanding need to be the priority—not just putting these problems on a list, but devoting money and time to solving them.

Funding is needed to collect evidence on what needs to be done. Wood showed us a system for standardizing drug labels—the universal medication schedule, or UMS. That was courageous leadership. Many at this conference said it would be good to obtain evidence about this approach. Obtaining evidence requires funding, but we need to be careful to identify what evidence we need.

Do we really need evidence of improved adherence to move forward with a standardized drug label? That is hard to get. On the other hand, we are good at measuring comprehension. It is logical that if one cannot comprehend the instructions on a drug label, one is most likely not to adhere to those instructions. Therefore, a good first step is evidence of improved comprehension, which we hope will then lead to improved adherence.

Someone spoke today about the idea that clinical trials could use a standardized schedule for administration of medications. That is an exciting idea, and Goldhammer said it was something worth looking at. Another exciting idea is for the Department of Veterans Affairs to introduce a standardized label and look at the effects.

Several people raised the issue of the cost of introducing a standardized label. We are currently spending a great deal on treating adverse drug events (ADEs), and we are going to be spending more if we do not address the current problems. Treating ADEs costs a lot, perhaps more than trying to fix the problem of drug labeling.

Many today said that drug labeling is only one issue in the complexity surrounding patient understanding and use of medications. That is true. Certainly counseling, better written information, and effective translations are also important. But change must start somewhere. The drug label is the primary source patients turn to for instructions on how to take their medications, so start with that. Improve the drug label.

Stopping once the drug label is changed is not an option. What is done with the drug label can be used to address such issues as translation into other languages. Physician and pharmacist counseling are also important components. But with a standardized label, a standard way of taking medication, patient counseling may benefit.

It is time to do a better job for our patients.

References

AAOS (American Academy of Orthopaedic Surgeons). 2007. *Discrepancy in healthcare utiliza-tion: Is more better in orthopaedic surgery?* http://www.aaos.org/news/bulletin/jun07/reimbursement2.asp (accessed December 4, 2007).

AAP (American Academy of Pediatrics). 2005. *Medication reconciliation.* http://www.aap.org/visit/MedicationReconciliationWebcast.ppt (accessed November 28, 2007).

ACPF (American College of Physicians Foundation). 2007. *Improving prescription drug con-tainer labeling in the United States: A health literacy and medication safety initiative.* Wash-ington, D.C.: ACPF.

APhA (American Pharmacists Association Foundation). 2007. *Diabetes ten city challenge.* http://www.aphafoundation.org/Programs/Diabetes_Ten_City_Challenge/ (accessed December 4, 2007).

Budnitz, D.S. 2007. *Drug safety in ambulatory care: Where is the patient?* PowerPoint presenta-tion at the Institute of Medicine Workshop on Changing Prescription Medication Use Container Instructions to Improve Health Literacy and Medication Safety.

Budnitz, D.S., and P.L. Layde. 2007. Outpatient drug safety: New steps in an old direction. *Pharmacoepidemiol Drug Saf* 16(2):160-165.

Budnitz, D.S., D.A. Pollack, K.N. Weidenback, A.B. Mendelsohn, T.J. Schroeder, and J.L. Annest. 2006. National surveillance of emergency department visits for outpatient adverse drug events. *JAMA* 296:1858-1866.

Davis, T.C., M.S. Wolf, P.F. Bass, M. Middlebrooks, E. Kennan, D.W. Baker, C.L. Bennett, R. Durazo-Arvizu, S. Savory, and R.M. Parker. 2006a. Low literacy impairs comprehen-sion of prescription drug warning labels. *J Gen Intern Med* 21:847-851.

Davis, T.C., M.S. Wolf, P.F. Bass, J.A. Thompson, H.H. Tilson, M. Neuberger, and R.M. Parker. 2006b. Literacy and misunderstanding prescription drug labels. *Ann Intern Med* 145:887-894.

Davis, T.C., M.S. Wolf, and R. Parker. 2007. *To err really is human: Misunderstanding medication labels.* PowerPoint presentation at the Institute of Medicine Workshop on Changing Prescription Medication Use Container Instructions to Improve Health Literacy and Medication Safety.

FDA (Food and Drug Administration). 2006. *Guidance, useful written consumer medication information (CMI)*. http://www.fda.gov/cder/guidance/7139fnl.htm (accessed November 15, 2007).

Federal Register, Vol. 70, No. 214, Monday November 7, 2005, page 67571, 42 CFR Part 423 Medicare. *Program: E-Prescribing and the Prescription Drug Program*; Final Rule.

Geographic.org. 2007. *Top 10 GDP countries 2000-2050*. http://www.photius.com/rankings/gdp_2050_projection.html (accessed December 4, 2007).

IOM (Institute of Medicine). 2007. *Preventing medication errors*. Washington, D.C.: The National Academies Press.

KFF (Kaiser Family Foundation). 2007. *Prescription drug trends*. http://www.kff.org/rxdrugs/upload/3057_06.pdf (accessed December 4, 2007).

NAAL (National Assessment of Adult Literacy). 2005. *A first look at the literacy of America's adults in the 21st century*. Washington, D.C.: National Center for Education Statistics.

PC Magazine. 2007. *Definition of HL7*. http://www.pcmag.com/encyclopedia_term/0,2542,t=HL7&i=44294,00.asp (accessed December 4, 2007).

Shrank, W.H., J. Agnew-Blais, N.K. Choudhry, M.S. Wolf, A.S. Kesselheim, J. Avorn, and P. Shekelle. 2007. The variability and quality of medication container labels. *Arch Intern Med* 167(16).

Wolf, M.S., T.C. Davis, W. Shrank, M. Neuberger, and R.M. Parker. 2006a. A critical review of FDA-approved Medication Guides. *Pat Educ Counsel* 62:316-322.

Wolf, M.S., T.C. Davis, P.F. Bass, H. Tilson, and R.M. Parker. 2006b. Misunderstanding prescription drug warning labels among patients with low literacy. *Am J Health System Pharm* 63:1048-1055.

Wolf, M.S., T.C. Davis, W. Shrank, D.N. Rapp, P.F. Bass, U.M. Connor, M. Clayman, and R.M. Parker. 2007. To err is human: Patient misinterpretations of prescription drug label instructions. *Pat Educ Counsel* 67:293-300.

Wood, A.J.J. 2007. *Simplifying medication scheduling: Can we confuse patients less?* PowerPoint presentation at the Institute of Medicine Workshop on Changing Prescription Medication Use Container Instructions to Improve Health Literacy and Medication Safety.

Zhan, C., I. Arispe, E. Kelley, T. Ding, C.W. Burt, J. Shinogle, and D. Stryer. 2005. Ambulatory care visits for treating adverse drug effects in the United States, 1995-2001. *Jt Comm J Qual Patient Saf* 31:372-378.

Appendix A

Workshop Agenda

**Changing Prescription Medication Use
Container Instructions to Improve
Health Literacy and Medication Safety**

**October 12, 2007
8:30 a.m. – 5:30 p.m.
Room 100**

**Keck Center of the National Academies
500 Fifth Street, NW
Washington, DC 20001**

8:30 – 8:40	Welcome and Opening Remarks **Moderator: George Isham, M.D., M.S.** Chair, Institute of Medicine Roundtable on Health Literacy Medical Director and Chief Health Officer HealthPartners
8:40 – 9:00	Drug Safety in Ambulatory Care—Where Is the Patient? **Dan Budnitz, M.D., M.P.H.** Medical Officer Division of Healthcare Quality Promotion Coordinating Center for Infectious Diseases, CDC
9:00 – 9:15	To Err Is Human: The Role of Health Literacy in Patient Care **Terry C. Davis, Ph.D.** Professor of Medicine and Pediatrics Louisiana State University Health Sciences Center

9:15 – 9:45	Findings of the ACP Foundation White Paper on Drug Labeling **Michael Wolf, Ph.D., M.P.H.** Assistant Professor of Preventive Medicine Feinberg School of Medicine, Northwestern University
9:45 – 10:00	Discussion of Morning Presentations
10:00 – 10:30	Simplification of Drug Dosing Times: Can We Confuse Patients Less? A Proposal for Standardization **Alastair J. J. Wood, M.D., F.A.C.P.** Managing Director Symphony Capital LLC
10:30 – 11:30	Panel I: Federal Agency Reaction to Prescription Use Instruction Standardization **Cindy Brach, M.P.P.** Senior Health Policy Researcher Agency for Healthcare Research and Quality **Nancy Ostrove, Ph.D.** Senior Advisor for Risk Communication, Office of Planning, Office of the Commissioner, Food and Drug Administration **Virginia Torrise, Pharm.D.** Deputy Chief Consultant for Pharmacy Benefits Management Department of Veterans Affairs
11:30 – 12:45	Panel II: Pharmacy Reaction to Prescription Use Instruction Standardization **Alan Goldhammer, Ph.D.** Deputy Vice President, Regulatory Affairs PhRMA **Darren K. Townzen, R.Ph., M.B.A.** Director of Pharmacy Systems Wal-Mart **Gerald McEvoy, Pharm.D.** Assistant Vice President of Drug Information American Society of Health-System Pharmacists **William Ellis, R.Ph., M.S.** Chief Executive Officer American Pharmacists Association Foundation
12:45 – 1:30	Lunch Break

1:30 – 2:40	Panel IIIa: Other Stakeholder Reaction to Prescription Use Instruction Standardization: Physicians and Patients
	William Dolan, M.D.
	   Board Member
	   American Medical Association
	Albert Wu, M.D., M.P.H.
	   Professor of Health Policy and Management
	   Bloomberg School of Public Health, Johns Hopkins University
	William Bullman, M.A.M.
	   Executive Vice President
	   National Council on Patient Information and Education
	Linda Weiss, Ph.D.
	   Researcher
	   Center for Urban Epidemiologic Studies
	   New York Academy of Medicine
	Mara Youdelman, J.D., L.L.M.
	   Staff Attorney
	   National Health Law Program

2:40 – 3:10	Panel IIIb: Other Stakeholder Reaction to Prescription Use Instruction Standardization: Educators of Pharmacists and Physicians
	Mary Ann F. Kirkpatrick, Ph.D.
	   Associate Dean for Student Affairs
	   Shenandoah University Bernard J. Dunn School of Pharmacy
	   American Association of Colleges of Pharmacy
	Merrill Egorin, M.D.
	   Professor of Medicine and Pharmacology
	   University of Pittsburgh School of Medicine
	   Co-Director, Molecular Therapeutics/Drug Discovery Program
	   University of Pittsburgh Cancer Institute
	   AAMC, Expert Panel on Education in Safe and Effective
	   Prescribing Practices

3:10 – 3:30	Break

3:30 – 4:45	Panel IV: What Would It Take to Move Toward Prescription Use Instruction Standardization?
	Roger Williams, M.D.
	   Executive Vice President
	   Chief Executive Officer
	   United States Pharmacopeia
	Darren K. Townzen, R.Ph., M.B.A.
	   Director of Pharmacy Systems
	   Wal-Mart
	   National Council for Prescription Drug Programs, Inc.
	Susan Johnson, Pharm.D., Ph.D.
	   Associate Director of the Office of Nonprescription Products
	   Food and Drug Administration
	Vanessa Cajina, M.P.A.
	   Regional Networks Coordinator
	   Latino Coalition for a Healthy California

4:45 – 5:30	Summary and Discussion Closng Remarks **Ruth Parker, M.D.** Associate Professor of Medicine, Emory University

Appendix B

Biosketches of the Workshop Speakers

Cindy Brach, M.P.P., is a senior health policy researcher at the Agency for Healthcare Research and Quality (AHRQ). She is AHRQ's lead on cultural competence and sits on a number of cultural competence advisory groups. In addition to her own cultural competence research, she has overseen the development of guides to assist health plans in implementing culturally and linguistically appropriate services and a research agenda for cultural competence in health care. Currently Ms. Brach is spearheading AHRQ's health literacy activities, coordinating AHRQ's work in developing measures and improving the evidence base, and integrating health literacy activities throughout AHRQ's portfolios.

Daniel Budnitz, M.D., M.P.H., is a medical officer with the Division of Healthcare Quality Promotion, Centers for Disease Control and Prevention (CDC), where he directs projects to monitor medication safety. His primary activity is directing and managing the National Electronic Injury Surveillance System–Cooperative Adverse Drug Event Surveillance Project. Dr. Budnitz has also worked to develop public health data standards and public health responses to disease outbreaks, terrorism, and natural disasters.

Dr. Budnitz received a B.A. (Government) from Harvard University, and an M.D. and M.P.H. (Epidemiology) from Emory University. After completing residency training in internal medicine at the Hospital of the University of Pennsylvania, he served as an epidemic intelligence service officer with CDC's Injury Center. He currently is a commander in the U.S.

Public Health Service and, as clinical assistant professor of internal medicine, Emory University, he is a practicing, board-certified internist.

William Bullman, M.A.M., joined the staff of the National Council on Patient Information and Education (NCPIE) in 1985, assuming staff leadership in 1995. Under his guidance, in 1995 NCPIE produced two authoritative resources on prescription medication adherence: *Prescription Medicine Adherence: A Review of the Baseline of Knowledge* and *Topical Bibliography on Prescription Medicine Adherence.* The Council also developed a series of provider- and setting-specific *Recommendations for Action to Advance Prescription Medicine Adherence.* In 1996 the Council collaborated with the American Medical Association (AMA) on the development of AMA's *Guidelines for Physicians for Counseling Patients About Prescription Medications in the Ambulatory Setting.* In 2000 Mr. Bullman, representing NCPIE, collaborated with the Food and Drug Administration's (FDA's) Center for Drug Evaluation and Research on the organization and implementation of the *Cyber-Smart Safety Coalition.* He also coordinated the development of NCPIE's "Talk About Prescriptions" Month (annually in October) and managed the annual national awareness campaign from 1986 to 1995.

Prior to joining NCPIE, Mr. Bullman served from 1979 to 1984 as community program development specialist with the National High Blood Pressure Education Program under a contract to Kappa Systems, Inc., from the Heart, Lung, and Blood Institute of the National Institutes of Health. He also served, from 1972 to 1978, as administrator for the Rockville Community Clinic in Rockville, Maryland.

Mr. Bullman received a B.A. from the University of Maryland in College Park and an M.A.M. from George Washington University in Washington, D.C.

Vanessa Cajina, M.P.A., coordinates and organizes regionally based advocacy efforts for the Latino Coalition for a Healthy California (LCHC). By engaging local leaders, LCHC has built a strong network of community-based organizations throughout California that take an active role in state policy and legislation. LCHC is California's only statewide organization that focuses specifically on Latino health by engaging in policy development, community education, and research. Focus areas include access to health care, reducing health disparities, and community health. LCHC has led the state in providing the baselines for cultural and linguistic standards in California's Medicaid program, as well as legislation and research to prevent childhood obesity and increase the number of Latinos working in the health professions.

Prior to joining LCHC, Ms. Cajina coordinated a county program to increase outreach, enrollment, retention, and utilization efforts for California's Medicaid and SCHIP programs and was part of the design panel for a county program to provide universal children's health insurance. She also oversees LCHC's legislation on prescription drugs and mental health. She is currently completing a master's of science in community development at the University of California, Davis.

Terry C. Davis, Ph.D., is professor of medicine and pediatrics at Louisiana State University Health Sciences Center in Shreveport (LSUHSC-S), where she also heads the Behavioral Science Unit of the Feist-Weiller Cancer Center. For the past 20 years, she has led an interdisciplinary team investigating the impact of patient literacy on health and health care. A pioneer in the field of health literacy, her seminal achievements include development of the Rapid Estimate of Adult Literacy in Medicine (REALM), the most widely used literacy test in health care settings, and production of videotapes that have personalized the problem of low health literacy.

Dr. Davis chaired Louisiana's statewide Health Literacy Task Force, the first legislatively mandated health literacy group in the nation. She currently serves on the master faculty of the American Medical Association's (AMA's) Train-the-Trainer Health Literacy Curriculum and is a member of the Healthy People 2010 Health Literacy/Health Communication Section and the Food and Drug Administration's (FDA's) Drug Safety and Risk Management Advisory Committee.

Dr. Davis has published more than 90 articles and book chapters related to health literacy, health communication, and preventive medicine. As director of the doctor/patient communication course at LSUHSC and as a frequent speaker at national conferences, she has integrated her research findings into practical lessons for medical students and residents, as well as practicing physicians, pharmacists, and nurses.

Dr. Davis, together with investigators at the University of North Carolina and the University of California at San Francisco, developed and tested a diabetes self-management guide funded by the American College of Physicians Foundation (ACPF), which has distributed more than 400,000 copies to our nation's physicians. She was recently awarded National Institutes of Health (NIH) funding for a five-year Health Literacy Intervention to improve cancer screening in Louisiana Federally Qualified Health Clinics. She is currently working with faculty at Northwestern University and Emory University to improve patient comprehension of medication labels. This research has received significant media notice by the *New York Times* and *USA Today*, NPR, CBS, ABC, and the BBC.

William Dolan, M.D., currently serves on the AMA-BOT Awards and Nominations Committee, the Group Practice Advisory Committee, the Task Force on Quality, Safety and Electronic Health Records, and the Health

System Reform Task Force. In addition, he is also on the AMA Council on Ethical and Judicial Affairs.

As a lead physician in a well-publicized class action suit against managed care companies, Dr. Dolan helped win $140 million in payments for New York physicians. More important, the lawsuit resulted in widespread reform of oppressive institutionalized business practices that had frustrated New York physicians for many years. As president of the Medical Society of the State of New York (MSSNY) and chairman of its board of trustees, Dr. Dolan was instrumental in leading the society into the 21st century as a founding member of the MSSNY Strategic Planning Task Force. The MSSNY Young Physicians Section also recognized Dr. Dolan for his leadership in championing issues of importance to younger physicians.

A practicing orthopedic surgeon and clinical professor at the University of Rochester, New York, Dr. Dolan was a member of Gov. George Pataki's Health Care Reform Act Quality Task Force and the committee to study proposed regulation of office-based surgery. Dr. Dolan also developed the Medical Quality Assurance Task Force, a statewide coalition of health care provider organizations that focus on eliminating errors in delivery of patient care. An active leader in the second-largest independent practice association in the United States, Dr. Dolan is well aware of physicians' fiscal, strategic, and practice management issues. He also is an active board member of the Medical Liability Mutual Insurance Company, the largest medical liability carrier in the country.

A native of Brooklyn, New York, Dr. Dolan attended Dalhousie University Medical School and obtained the M.D. cum laude with many honors, including Alpha Omega Alpha. He served as a lieutenant commander in the U.S. Navy.

Merrill J. Egorin, M.D., is codirector of the Molecular Therapeutics/Drug Discovery Program at the University of Pittsburgh Cancer Institute (UPCI) and a professor of medicine and pharmacology at the University of Pittsburgh School of Medicine.

Dr. Egorin's research focuses on rational development and application of antineoplastic agents. He serves as principal investigator on a National Cancer Institute-funded contract evaluating the pharmacokinetics, metabolism, and pharmacodynamics of antitumor agents being considered for clinical trials and is the co–principal investigator of a National Cancer Institute–funded cooperative agreement for conducting Phase I studies at UPCI. Key concepts regularly addressed in Dr. Egorin's research involve the pharmacokinetic and pharmacodynamic relationships of investigational and licensed antineoplastic agents and how those relationships can be assessed and modeled.

Dr. Egorin received his M.D. and training in internal medicine from the Johns Hopkins University School of Medicine and Hospital. Early in his career, he joined the Baltimore Cancer Research Center, then part of the National Cancer Institute. In 1981 he became a staff physician at the University of Maryland Hospital, where he rose to the position of professor of medicine, pharmacology and experimental therapeutics, and oncology. Dr. Egorin was recruited to UPCI in 1998 to lead its clinical and preclinical pharmacology activities.

Dr. Egorin's professional affiliations include a fellowship in the American College of Physicians and memberships in the American Association for Cancer Research, the American Society for Clinical Oncology, the American Society for Clinical Pharmacology and Therapeutics, and the American Society for Pharmacology and Experimental Therapeutics. He serves on the editorial boards of several medical journals and is editor-in-chief of *Cancer Chemotherapy and Pharmacology*. Dr. Egorin has authored or coauthored numerous book chapters and more than 175 articles in peer-reviewed journals.

William Ellis, R.Ph., M.S., is the executive director and chief executive officer of the American Pharmacists Association (APhA) Foundation. The APhA Foundation, headquartered in Washington, D.C., is a nonprofit organization affiliated with APhA, the national professional society of pharmacists in the United States. The APhA Foundation has expertise in designing programs that seek to create a new medication use system in the United States where patients, pharmacists, physicians, and other health care providers collaborate to dramatically improve the cost and quality of consumer health outcomes. Mr. Ellis oversees all APhA Foundation activities, including awards programs, research initiatives, and related consulting services. He serves on the Healthcare Practitioner Advisory Council of the National Committee on Quality Assurance, and represents APhA on the National Quality Forum. Mr. Ellis received his B.S. in pharmacy from the Philadelphia College of Pharmacy and Science (1985), completed a one-year postgraduate program in association management, and has an M.S. in health education from St. Joseph's University (1994).

Alan Goldhammer, Ph.D., is deputy vice president for regulatory affairs at the Pharmaceutical Research and Manufacturers of America (PhRMA). In this position he manages activities of the Regulatory Affairs Coordinating Committee, maintaining a liaison with the Food and Drug Administration on important drug regulatory issues.

Prior to coming to PhRMA, Dr. Goldhammer was executive director, technical affairs, for the Biotechnology Industry Organization (BI). He also served as regulatory affairs consultant to the International Food

Biotechnology Council, a Washington-based organization that developed scientific criteria for assuring the safety of foods produced through biotechnology.

Before joining the BI, Dr. Goldhammer was a senior staff fellow in the Clinical Endocrinology Branch at the National Institutes of Health. He held an NIH postdoctoral fellowship at Cornell University. He has a B.A. in chemistry from the University of California, Santa Barbara, and a Ph.D. in biological chemistry from Indiana University. He is a member of the American Chemical Society and the American Association for the Advancement of Science.

George Isham, M.D., M.S., is medical director and chief health officer for HealthPartners. He is responsible for Quality and Utilization Management, chairs the Benefits Committee, and leads Partners for Better Health, a program and strategy for improving member health. Before his current position, he was medical director of MedCenters Health Plan in Minneapolis. In the late 1980s, he was executive director of University Health Care, an organization affiliated with the University of Wisconsin–Madison.

Dr. Isham received his M.S. in preventive medicine/administrative medicine at the University of Wisconsin–Madison and his M.D. from the University of Illinois. He served his internship and residency in internal medicine at the University of Wisconsin Hospital and Clinics in Madison. His practice experience as a primary care physician included 8 years at the Freeport Clinic in Freeport, Illinois, and 3½ years as clinical assistant professor in medicine at the University of Wisconsin.

HealthPartners is a consumer-governed Minnesota health plan, formed through the 1992 affiliation of Group Health, Inc., and MedCenters Health Plan. HealthPartners is a large managed health care organization in Minnesota, representing nearly 800,000 members. Group Health, founded in 1957, is a network of staff medical and dental centers located throughout the Twin Cities. MedCenters, founded in 1972, is a network of contracted physicians serving members through affiliated medical and dental centers.

Susan Johnson, Pharm.D., Ph.D., received her Pharm.D. and Ph.D. in clinical pharmacy from Purdue University and came to the Center for Drug Evaluation and Research (CDER) of the U.S. Food and Drug Administration in 1990. She was a clinical reviewer in the Division of Pulmonary and Allergy Drug Products for 10 years, before moving to CDER's Review Standards Staff in 2000 and then to the Office of New Drugs Immediate Office in 2002. Since 2004, Susan has served as the associate director of the Office of Nonprescription Products and acting director of the Division of Nonprescription Regulation Development.

Mary Ann F. Kirkpatrick, Ph.D., received a B.S. in pharmacy from the University of North Carolina at Chapel Hill and an M.S. in gerontology and a Ph.D. in urban services from Virginia Commonwealth University (VCU). Dr. Kirkpatrick has practiced in retail and hospital pharmacies and taught compounding and dispensing in the School of Pharmacy at VCU for 20 years prior to becoming the associate dean for student affairs in the Shenandoah University Bernard J. Dunn School of Pharmacy.

She is a coauthor of the Virginia Medication Management Training program required for all medication aides working in licensed adult care facilities in Virginia and has also engaged in research investigating the readability of patient drug monographs.

Dr. Kirkpatrick has received several awards for her research, service and teaching, including an American Society on Aging Research Award (1998), the Virginia Department of Social Services Outstanding Service Award (1993), the VCU School of Pharmacy Teaching Excellence Award (1991), and the Virginia Geriatric Education Center Outstanding Service Award (2001).

Gerald McEvoy, Pharm.D., is assistant vice president of drug information at the American Society of Health-System Pharmacists (ASHP) and editor-in-chief of *AHFS Drug Information,* ASHP's federally recognized drug compendium. He has established expertise in evidence-based medical publishing, focusing on rational drug therapy and safe medication use, and has led ASHP's distinguished drug information publishing activities for over 25 years.

Dr. McEvoy serves on the board of directors of the National Council on Patient Information and Education (NCPIE), has testified before and advised the U.S. Food and Drug Administration on medication safety communication issues involving consumers, and has spoken internationally on the provision of safe medication use information to consumers.

Before joining ASHP, Dr. McEvoy was on the faculty of Creighton University's School of Pharmacy in Omaha, Nebraska. He obtained both his B.S. and Pharm.D. in pharmacy from Duquesne University in Pittsburgh and completed a hospital residency at Mercy Hospital in Pittsburgh.

Nancy Ostrove, Ph.D., is senior advisor for risk communication in the Office of Planning in Food and Drug Administration's (FDA's) Office of the Commissioner. She is the agency lead in assessing FDA's risk communication approaches and programs, developing risk communication strategies for the strategic priority area of improving patient and consumer safety, and identifying issues to be brought to the Risk Communication Advisory Committee.

Dr. Ostrove was with FDA's Center for Drug Evaluation and Research from 1989 until 2002, where she was deputy director and branch chief in the Division of Drug Marketing, Advertising, and Communications. Her work focused on research, consulting, and policy development related to communicating prescription drug information to health care professionals and consumers. Dr. Ostrove led the early development of FDA's "direct-to-consumer" (DTC) promotion policies. She also conducted the research and development of FDA's proposal to revise the format of prescription drug labeling to be more useful for prescribers. She was key in developing FDA's Medication Guide rules and in research assessing the private-sector effort to ensure that patients getting new prescription medicines receive useful written information about these medicines.

Dr. Ostrove received her Ph.D. in social psychology in 1976 from the University of Maryland at College Park and received postdoctoral training in medical psychology from the Uniformed Services University of the Health Sciences. She has taught undergraduate students and conducted applied psychological and marketing research for the private sector. From 2002 to 2003, Dr. Ostrove served as regulatory liaison for Eli Lilly and Company.

Virginia Torrise, Pharm.D., is the deputy chief consultant for Pharmacy Benefits Management (PBM) staff at the Department of Veterans Affairs. In the post, she serves as the chief operating officer for the PBM program. Before taking this position, she was the chief of the pharmacy service at the Greater Los Angeles VA health care system.

Darren K. Townzen, R.Ph., M.B.A., started his career with Wal-Mart in 1989 as a pharmacist in east Texas. He then moved to Bentonville, Arkansas, in 1995 to manage the drug database and other projects. His current responsibilities as director of pharmacy systems for Wal-Mart include systems project management and drug and insurance claim formats and billing.

Mr. Townzen graduated from Southwestern Oklahoma University at Weatherford in 1988 with a B.S. in pharmacy and obtained an M.B.A. from Webster University in 2006.

Linda Weiss, Ph.D., is a researcher in the Center for Urban Epidemiologic Studies at the New York Academy of Medicine (NYAM). She has a Ph.D. in cultural anthropology from Columbia University and has examined health care access issues among diverse populations including immigrants, people living with HIV/AIDS, the elderly, children, and substance users. She recently served as principal investigator on a study of the availability of translated medication information from New York City pharmacists and is currently directing a follow-up project focused on training pharmacists and conducting pilot interventions to improve access to multilingual medication instructions. Other current work includes participation in a study of the role of Asian immigrant institutions in HIV prevention and education, an examination of neighborhood predictors of health behaviors and health outcomes, and a multisite evaluation of programs to integrate opioid treatment into HIV primary care. Previous work at NYAM includes a study of language and other barriers to health insurance and health care for children in immigrant families, a study of the ethical responsibilities of hospital trustees, and an evaluation of programs to support adherence to HIV medications.

Roger Williams, M.D., has been the executive vice president and chief executive officer of the United States Pharmacopeia (USP) since April 2000. Working with a staff of nearly 400, Dr. Williams provides strategic leadership for USP at the direction of USP's board of trustees. He also serves as chair of the Council of Experts, USP's scientific body, which continuously revises the United States Pharmacopeia and National Formulary (USP–NF).

Since joining USP, Dr. Williams has led a reengineering effort designed to ensure that USP's products and services meet the needs of its constituencies. These constituencies include practitioners and patients/consumers who seek safe, effective, and good-quality therapeutic products, as well as pharmaceutical manufacturers, compounding professionals, and many other stakeholders. Dr. Williams has reorganized the structure of the Council of Experts, brought focus to its science-based decisions, and aligned USP's efforts with other pharmacopeias throughout the world. He has established stakeholder forums that promote communication with and input from pharmaceutical and dietary supplement manufacturers, compounding professionals, patient safety advocates, and USP's membership.

Dr. Williams is USP's lead representative for international activities and outreach efforts to the many professional groups and societies who share USP's public health mission. The strength of USP's public programs has allowed USP to expand its public health mission both nationally and internationally. USP established a site in India in 2006 and in 2005 opened a sales office in Basel, Switzerland. The USP–NF was published in Spanish in 2005.

Michael Wolf, Ph.D., M.P.H., is an assistant professor in the Center for Healthcare Studies at Northwestern University's Feinberg School of Medicine. He is a faculty fellow at the Institute for Health Services Research and Policy Studies and on senior staff for the Chicago VA Healthcare System's Midwest Center for Health Services and Policy Research. Dr. Wolf is an alumnus of Valparaiso University and earned his Ph.D. at the University of Illinois and his M.P.H. at Northwestern University. Prior to his current position at the center, Dr. Wolf received postdoctoral training in health services research at the Institute for Health Services Research and Policy Studies, which culminated in his receiving the Pfizer Health Literacy Initiative Scholar's Award. He is also a member of the Robert H. Lurie Comprehensive Cancer Center and recently received the Coleman Foundation Young Investigator Fellowship for conducting cancer research. Dr. Wolf's research interests focus on the reduction of health disparities, health communication, HIV/AIDS and cancer prevention, and health promotion.

Alastair J. J. Wood, M.D., F.A.C.P., received his M.D. from St. Andrew's University and Dundee Medical School in Scotland. He joined the faculty at Vanderbilt University School of Medicine in 1978, where he became tenured professor of both medicine and pharmacology and attending physician at Vanderbilt Medical School. He was assistant vice chancellor for clinical research (1999–2004) and associate dean, Vanderbilt Medical School (2004–2006), before being appointed emeritus professor of medicine and emeritus professor of pharmacology in 2006. His current academic appointments are professor of medicine and professor of pharmacology at Weill Cornell Medical College, New York.

Dr. Wood is a member of many societies and has received numerous honors, notably election to membership in the Institute of Medicine of the National Academy of Sciences, the American Association of Physicians, and the American Society for Clinical Investigation. He is honorary fellow, American Gynecological and Obstetrical Society (AGOS), and has fellowship in the American College of Physicians, the Royal College of Physicians of London, and the Royal College of Physicians of Edinburgh. He was the 2005 recipient of the Rawls-Palmer Award from the American Society for Pharmacology and Experimental Therapeutics in recognition of "Drug investigation that brings the effects of modern drug research to the care of patients."

Dr. Wood has served on a number of editorial boards. He was a member of the *New England Journal of Medicine* editorial board from 2004 to 2006; he was the drug therapy editor of the *New England Journal of Medicine* from 1985 to 2004; and he is on the editorial board of *Clinical Pharmacology and Therapeutics* and the *Scientist*. He has previously served on the editorial boards of the *British Journal of Clinical Pharmacology* and *Biopharmaceutics and Drug Disposition*. He authored a chapter in Harrison's *Principles of Internal Medicine* on adverse drug reactions for the 9th through the 15th editions.

Dr. Wood was chairman of the Food and Drug Administration's (FDA's) Nonprescription Drugs Advisory Committee until 2006 and chaired the 2005 FDA Advisory Committee on Cox-2 inhibitors. He previously served as a member of the FDA's Cardiovascular and Renal Advisory Committee and Nonprescription Drugs Advisory Committee. He has been both a member and chair of NIH study sections and has served in a similar capacity for various philanthropic grant-giving bodies. He has served as a director of pharmaceutical companies, including Antigenics, Symphony Neurodevelopment, and Symphony Evolution. He has also served as a consultant to pharmaceutical companies, investors, and academic institutions. He has provided congressional testimony and directly interacted with and advised senior White House officials, legislators, and the secretary of health on matters related to public health. He is a frequent commentator in the national press on issues related to medicine and pharmaceuticals.

His research interests have been focused on understanding the mechanisms for interindividual variability in drug response, with a particular focus on the molecular genetics of adrenergic receptors, ethnic differences in drug response, vascular response, and the genetics of drug metabolism. His research has been continuously funded by the National Institutes of Health and has resulted in over 280 articles, reviews, and editorials.

Albert W. Wu, M.D., M.P.H., is an practicing internist and professor of health policy and management at the Johns Hopkins Bloomberg School of Public Health, with joint appointments in epidemiology, international health, medicine, and surgery. He received his B.A. and M.D. from Cornell University and completed an internal medicine residency at the Mount Sinai Hospital and University of California (UC) San Diego. He was a Robert Wood Johnson clinical scholar at UC San Francisco, and received an M.P.H. from UC Berkeley. His research and teaching focus on patient outcomes and quality of care. He has studied the handling of medical errors since 1998 and has published influential papers including "Do house officers learn from their mistakes" in *JAMA* in 1991; "To tell the truth—ethical and practical issues in disclosing medical mistakes to patients" in the *Journal of General Internal Medicine;* and "Medical error: the second victim" in the *BMJ.* He was co–principal investigator of an Agency for Healthcare Research and Quality (AHRQ)-funded grant to develop a web-based incident reporting system for intensive care units. He is principal investigator of the AHRQ-funded Johns Hopkins DEcIDE Center to conduct rapid, policy-relevant studies of comparative effectiveness. He is studying video vignettes of disclosures to patient and their families and has developed an award-winning educational video on disclosure titled "Removing insult from injury: disclosing adverse events." He was a member of the Institute of Medicine Committee on Identifying and Preventing Medication Errors and is a member of the Hopkins Quality and Safety Research Group. He is senior advisor to the World Alliance for Patient Safety.

Mara Youdelman, J.D., L.L.M., has been a staff attorney in the National Health Law Program's Washington, D.C., office for over 4 years. She works on issues such as language access, civil rights, Medicaid, and racial and ethnic disparities in health care. She received her J.D. from Boston University School of Law and her L.L.M. from Georgetown University Law Center.

Appendix C

ACP White Paper

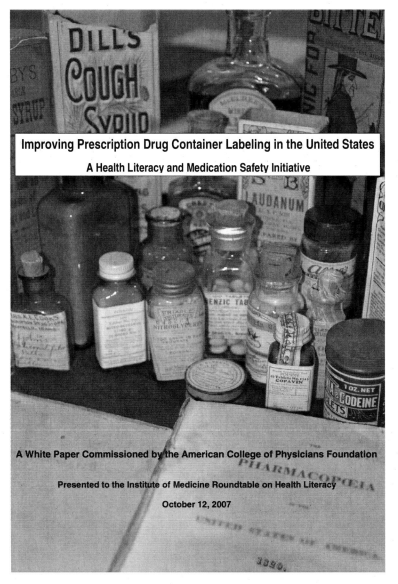

Improving Prescription Drug Container Labeling in the United States

A Health Literacy and Medication Safety Initiative

A White Paper Commissioned by the American College of Physicians Foundation

Presented to the Institute of Medicine Roundtable on Health Literacy

October 12, 2007

REPORT PRESENTED ON BEHALF OF THE ACPF MEDICATION LABELING TECHNICAL ADVISORY BOARD

Committee Co-Chairs:

Michael S. Wolf, PhD, MPH Feinberg School of Medicine, Northwestern University

Ruth M. Parker, MD Emory University School of Medicine

Members:

Carolyn Clancy, MD Agency for Healthcare Research and Quality

Frank Frederico, RPh Institute for Healthcare Improvement

Charles Ganley, MD Food and Drug Administration

William H. Shrank, MD MSHS Brigham and Women's Hospital; Harvard Medical School

Scott Smith, PhD PharmD Agency for Healthcare Research and Quality

Roger Williams, MD U.S. Pharmacopeia

Alastair Wood, MD Symphony Capital, LLC

Albert Wu, MD MPH Johns Hopkins Bloomberg School of Public Health

ACPF Staff:

Robert L. Harnsberger, MBA, VP/COO American College of Physicians Foundation

Jean A. Krause, EVP/CEO American College of Physicians Foundation

Acknowledgments:

John Swann, PhD Food and Drug Administration

Diane Wendt Smithsonian Institution

Special Thanks:

Stacy Cooper Bailey, MPH Northwestern University

Kara Jacobson, MPH Emory University

CONTENTS

EXECUTIVE SUMMARY

According to the Institute of Medicine (IOM) 2006 report, *Preventing Medication Errors,* more than half a million adverse drug events (ADEs) occur in the United States each year in outpatient settings. Problems with prescription drug (Rx) labeling were cited as the cause of a large proportion of outpatient medication errors and ADEs, as patients may unintentionally misuse a prescribed medicine due to improper understanding of instructions. Recent health literacy research has highlighted the alarmingly high prevalence of patients misunderstanding seemingly simple instructions and warnings placed on Rx container labels. The elderly, those with limited literacy skills, and individuals managing multiple medication regimens were found to be at greater risk for making errors in interpreting container label instructions.

The ability to understand Rx container label instructions is critical, both as health literacy and medication safety concerns. This is especially true since other sources of patient medication information are insufficient. Prior studies have found that physicians and pharmacists frequently miss opportunities to adequately counsel patients on newly prescribed medicines. Other supplementary sources, such as patient information leaflets and Medication Guides dispensed with the prescribed medicine are too complex and written at a reading level unsuitable for the majority of patients to comprehend. As a result, these materials are often ignored. While all of these sources are best viewed as a system of patient information, the Rx container label is particularly important as it is often the sole source of specific instructions received and repeatedly used by patients on how to self-administer medicines.

Despite its potential value, there are clear problems with Rx container labels. Minimal standards and regulations exist regarding their content and format, and Rx labels can vary by dispensing pharmacy. Specific dosage instructions on the container label are dependent on what the prescribing physician writes, as well as how the pharmacist interprets these instructions. While the format and content of Rx container labels may differ between and within local and national pharmacies, all share the common attribute of being unnecessarily complex and not offering a patient-friendly interface. Instead, the greatest emphasis is placed on provider-directed content.

This report reviews in detail the problem with Rx container labels in the United States. The "best practices" in drug container labeling are summarized. Recommendations are offered to guide medical and pharmacy practice, and related state and federal policy. The overall objective of this paper is to move forward a set of evidence-based, Rx container label standards that will minimize patient confusion and promote patient aware-

TABLE 1 Primary Findings

Finding 1	Inadequate patient understanding of prescription medication instructions and warnings is prevalent and a significant safety concern.
Finding 2	Lack of universal standards and regulations for medication labeling is a "root cause" for misunderstanding and medication error.
Finding 3	An evidence-based set of practices should guide all label content and format.
Finding 4	Instructions for use on the container label are especially important for patients and should be clear and concise. Language should be standardized to improve patient understanding for safe and effective use.
Finding 5	Drug labeling should be viewed as part of an integrated system of patient information. Improvements are needed beyond the container label, and other sources of consumer medication information should be targeted.
Finding 6	Health care providers are not adequately communicating to patients, either orally or in print, about prescribed medicines. More training is needed to promote best practices for writing prescriptions and counseling patients.
Finding 7	Support is necessary for research on drug labeling and to identify "best practices" for patient medication information.

ness of how to use a prescribed medicine safely and effectively, thereby reducing risk of medication error.

PROLOGUE

Since 2002, the American College of Physicians Foundation (ACPF) has sought to address the problem of limited health literacy by developing initiatives to mitigate the impact of this highly prevalent problem on health outcomes. The issue of inconsistent and confusing medication information and labeling soon became a primary target of the ACPF health literacy agenda. A few projects were commissioned by the ACPF, and informal activities were spearheaded to engage experts and stakeholders from academia, industry, and government. In September 2006, a meeting was held in Washington, D.C. to discuss the ACPF's medication labeling initiatives and to suggest next steps for ACPF. The overall objective of the meeting was to consolidate an understanding of the broad problem of inadequate patient understanding of medication labels, and to identify a specific course of action to improve drug labeling in the United States. The meeting served as a timely response to Institute of Medicine (IOM) reports, released in July and September 2006, which targeted medication error and drug safety, respectively. Participants at this meeting included national experts in health literacy, patient safety, pharmacology, and pharmacy policy and practice. The Agency for Healthcare Research and Quality (AHRQ), the Institute of Medicine (IOM), and the Food and Drug Administration (FDA) were represented.

Participants reviewed the nature and extent of the problems surrounding medication labeling, particularly for prescription drugs. Summaries were provided from the July 2006 IOM report, *Preventing Medication Errors,* the FDA over-the-counter (OTC) consumer education initiatives, an ACPF-commissioned medication labeling systematic literature review, and recent health literacy research studies. Herein, this white paper presents the ACPF perspective on the current prescription medication container labeling system, with a focus on improving the format, content, and dosage and use instructions on the container label.

PRESCRIPTION DRUG CONTAINER LABELING: A MEDICATION SAFETY CONCERN

Patient safety remains one of the most important objectives for health care providers and organizations.[1-5] Medication errors, in particular, are the most common form of mistakes that lead to patient injury, hospitalization, and death.[6-19] According to the recent IOM report, *Preventing Medication Errors,* approximately 1.5 million preventable adverse drug events occur each year; more than one third of these take place in outpatient settings at a cost approaching $1 billion annually.[20] Both physicians and patients identify this as an area of serious concern, as a growing number of adults self-administer prescription medicines each year. Errors in ambulatory care are likely to increase as patients are self-managing a greater number of prescription and over-the-counter (OTC) medications. Two thirds of all adults use prescription drugs, representing 16 percent ($73 billion) of all health care expenditures.[21] According to the Medical Expenditures Panel Survey (MEPS), the average number of prescription medications filled annually by adults in the United States increased between 1996 and 2003 from 7 to 10 prescriptions. Among adults over 65 years of age, the average number of prescriptions filled increased from 19 to 27 medicines during this same time period.[21] Further complicating the problem, elderly patients are cared for by an average of 8 different health providers, each of whom may use different instructions for the same dosing frequencies. A clear understanding of the existing failures has therefore been sought to reduce the potential for costly errors in the future.

There is a limited body of evidence detailing the possible causes of outpatient medication error. Attention to the causes of error has most often been directed to the role of the health care provider or the system in causing errors during the prescribing, ordering, dispensing or administering of a medicine.[1] This may be an appropriate focus for inpatient hospital or nursing home settings, where most studies investigating medication error have been conducted.[15-19] However, studies estimate that many outpatient medication errors occur when patients themselves fail to administer a medicine as intended.[6,7,13,14,22,23] For ambulatory care, the patient, rather than the provider, is ultimately responsible for correctly administering a medicine as prescribed. In this setting, the processes of quality control and monitoring of medication use shift from provider to patient.[14]

Given the formative role patients must play in promoting medication safety in outpatient settings, it is instructive to understand current processes that can help an individual learn how to use prescribed medicines appropriately. These include both verbal and written communication about taking medication; it is the tangible, written sources that comprise drug container labeling that are of special interest to this report. Figure 1 provides a breakdown of what specifically is meant by the broader term of "drug labeling." The prescription container label warrants special attention, as it often may be the only prescription drug information seen and used repeatedly by patients. As this report will detail, container labels for prescription drugs have been undervalued and neglected, despite their critical importance in conveying instructions for use to patients.

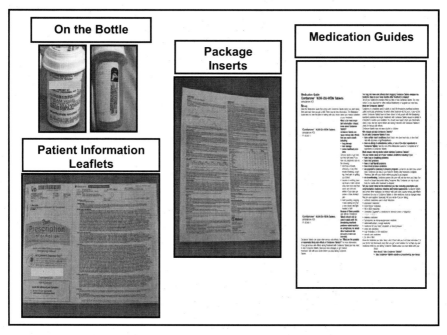

FIGURE 1 Components of drug labeling.

THE PATIENT PERSPECTIVE

The past 100 years have led to a fractured system of delivering adequate assurances of instructions for safe and effective use of prescription drugs to patients. In the past decade, the health literacy movement in the United States has placed greater attention on the responsibility of the health care system to support patients' ability to read, understand, and act on health information. Health literacy emphasizes the unique value of container labeling for prescription drugs as a patient source of essential health information, vital for drug safety and efficacy.

A Health Literacy Concern

Recent studies have highlighted limited health literacy as a potential risk factor for higher rates of outpatient medication error that are the result of improper dosing administration.[20,22,24] Health literacy, as defined by the IOM report *A Prescription to End Confusion* and accepted by the National Library of Medicine, is the "degree to which individuals have the capacity to obtain, process, and understand basic health information and services needed to make appropriate health decisions."[24] An estimated one third to one half of adults in the United States—as many as 90 million Americans—possess limited health literacy skills, and may have trouble understanding and acting on health materials. Information in less familiar print contexts, such as prescription container labels, may be confusing and more difficult to comprehend for less literate patients.[25]

According to the National Assessment of Adult Literacy (NAAL) of 2003, 14% of U.S. adults possess skills in the lowest level of prose and document literacy ("below basic"), and 22% are at the lowest level for quantitative literacy.[25] These individuals can perform only the most simple, concrete tasks associated with each of these domains. However, those with only "basic" literacy proficiency have limited abilities and are likely to be hindered in routine daily activities. Considering individuals with basic and below basic skills combined, as many as 34% to 55% of adults in the U.S. have limited literacy skills. Estimates are significantly higher among the elderly; 60% of individuals over the age of 65 have limited levels of prose and document literacy.[25]

Yet reading fluency and the full range of literacy skills are likely to vary with an individual's familiarity with the content of the text.[26-28] Health materials and encounters often use difficult and unfamiliar medical terms.[29] Therefore, the estimates of limited health literacy using the NAAL general literacy assessment may underestimate the problem. As a response to this concern, the NAAL 2003 included a health literacy assessment designed to measure respondents' abilities to locate and understand health-related information and services. The health literacy assessment reported average health literacy scores on a scale of 100 to 500, with 500 representing the highest possible score. The assessment also reported results by grouping respondents with similar scores into performance levels based on health literacy ability. The performance levels designated by the assessment were: below basic, basic, intermediary, and proficient.[30] Results from the health literacy assessment showed the average health literacy scores of Americans to be lower than the average general literacy scores of adults, as measured by the NAAL. Those over 65 years of age had a health literacy mean score of 214 (the lowest average score; threshold between below basic and basic proficiency) compared to a mean score of 256 for adults between the age of 25 and 39 (the highest average score).[30] The conclusion remains the same: millions of U.S. adults—especially the elderly—lack the health literacy skills that enable them to effectively use complex health materials and accomplish more challenging health-related tasks.

Sources of Patient Prescription Medication Information

The IOM *Health Literacy* report emphasized that the problem of limited health literacy cannot be viewed solely as a patient issue.[24] Rather, health literacy is a duality, reflecting both individual capability and the complexity of demands placed upon the individual by the health care system. This perspective is equally valid for medication labeling in the United States. While patients must have cognitive capacity and proficiency to read and understand labels, and apply dosage/usage instructions for proper medicine-taking behaviors, the manner in which the current health care system delivers necessary medication information to patients is inadequate. Understanding the sources available to patients and their deficits provides for a comprehensive picture of current health system failures and remedies. The existing continuum of sources of patient medication information begins at the moment a prescription is issued to the patient by the physician (see Figure 2). Physicians, with legal responsibilities to deliver instructions on proper medication use, have repeatedly been found to be ineffective in this role.[31-35] Research has shown physicians frequently miss opportunities to counsel their patients on how to self-administer their medicines.[31,34] Health literacy studies have also highlighted that many physicians do not communicate health and treatment information in a manner that can be understood by patients with limited literacy skills.[36-38] Written prescriptions will be passed on to patients, yet these are typically written with unfamiliar shorthand, often in Latin, and therefore of little use to patients.[1,39,40]

If the patient leaves the physician office without the knowledge needed to correctly implement the prescribed regimen, the pharmacist,

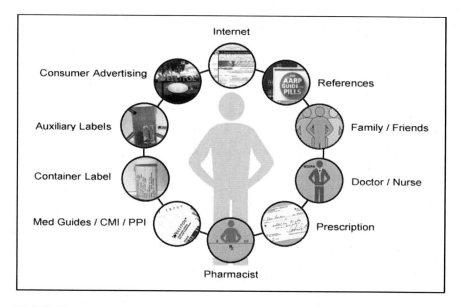

FIGURE 2 Sources of patient medication information.
NOTE: CMI = Consumer Medication Information; PPI = Patient Package Insert.

at the point of dispensing medicines, would be next in line to counsel patients. Studies have shown that pharmacists also often fail to orally communicate detailed information to patients to support their adherence with prescribed regimens.[32,33,35] The last opportunity for counseling is the container label and accompanying print materials (container label, patient package inserts, consumer medication information, Medication Guides), which have been found to be long, complex, and written at a level too difficult for a majority of patients, regardless of literacy level, to comprehend and use.[38,42-46]

Without accurate and available formal sources of information, individuals may seek out informal sources to learn about their medicines. Informal sources might include social networks (family, informal caregivers, friends), the internet and other reference materials. No assurances can be made to the quality, accuracy, or readability of the information provided within these sources, as their content is not regulated.[41,42,47-49]

Health Literacy and Medication Safety

Numerous studies have found limited health literacy to be significantly associated with a poorer understanding of medication names, indications, and instructions.[50-59] More recently, health literacy skills have been linked to requisite knowledge necessary for adherence to treatment regimens.[22,23,60] Recently, health literacy was specifically identified within a seminal report released by the National Council for Patient Information and Education (NCPIE).[61] The report refers to health literacy as a national concern with regard to patient understanding, safe use, and proper adherence to medication regimens.[61]

A current and well-publicized body of research has focused on the ability of patients to read, understand, and demonstrate instructions on prescription medication container labels.[22,23] This line of inquiry has also been supported by parallel work in human factors research, which has more broadly investigated similar measures, mostly among the elderly.[62-68] Davis et al. conducted a multi-site study among adults receiving primary care at community health centers and found a high prevalence of patients, especially those with limited literacy, misunderstanding seemingly simple dose instructions provided on the primary label of medication containers.[22] In this study, 46% of adults misunderstood at least one prescription container label they encountered. The problem extends to the auxiliary sticker labels that provide accompanying warnings and instructions for use of the medicine (see Figure 2).[23,60] Other studies demonstrated that over half (53%) of patients, especially those with limited literacy, had difficulty interpreting text and icons commonly used on auxiliary warning instructions.[23]

Beyond the container label, another recent study also found accompanying medication information materials that provide indications for use and precautions are not useful for most patients, particularly those with limited health literacy.[46] This includes consumer Medication Guides that are required by the FDA to accompany certain prescribed medicines that have been identified as having serious public health concerns.[69-75] Patients with limited health literacy were significantly more likely to report not having reviewed these materials. These findings are supported by earlier research studies that suggested consumer medication materials are too difficult for many patients to read.[76-77] As a result, the patient information leaflets that accompany many prescription medications may be ignored.

Patients with limited health literacy may possess less knowledge of how to take their medicines not only as a result of difficulty with medicine labeling, but due to more limited interactions with health care providers and use of fewer alternative sources of informational support (i.e., internet, reference guides).[78] Prior research found patients with limited literacy skills to be more likely to report their physician as their sole source of health information, including for medicines taken for a chronic disease. Individuals with limited literacy are also less likely to seek out information or ask for clarification during medical encounters as a result of feelings of shame and concern over stigma for their poor reading ability.[79-81]

A BROKEN SYSTEM

The problems associated with prescription container labeling are ultimately the result of an apparent lack of standards and regulatory oversight. This results in patients receiving medications with highly variable labels, which they frequently do not understand. This is an issue of patient safety and successful therapeutic outcomes. Current drug prescribing and dispensing practices allow for variability in container labels. A lack of integration among the existing health information systems that support an increasing number of prescribers and the majority of dispensing pharmacies also adds to labeling difficulties.

The Prescriber

The container label offers perhaps the only written documentation of dosage/usage instructions for the patient, which are imparted through the physician's prescription. In most pharmacies today, whatever the physician writes is what is transcribed onto the container label. Although there may be a finite number of ways a prescription can be written, the same dose and frequency schedule for a prescribed drug may be written in several different ways (i.e., every twelve hours, twice daily, in the morning and evening, at 8 am and 5 pm, etc.). Physicians also use a variety of Latin abbreviations to identify drug dose and frequency, rendering the prescription uninterpretable to most patients. This becomes especially problematic as many patients, especially the elderly, may have more than one health care provider prescribing medicine. It is unclear if physicians and other prescribing health care providers receive adequate training in writing prescriptions. Although electronic prescribing offers options for enhanced safety, it is still necessary to determine what physician prescribing notations optimize patients' safe and effective use of their medications.

The Dispensing Pharmacy

The contents of labels are also highly variable depending on which pharmacy a patient selects. In a recent study, data were gathered from identically written prescriptions filled for four commonly prescribed drugs (atorvastatin, alendronate, trimethoprim-sulfamethoxazole, ibuprofen) in 6 different pharmacies (2 chains, 2 independents, and 2 grocery stores) in 4 diverse cities.[82] Evaluation of the format of labels on filled prescriptions suggests that labels are not designed to optimize patient understanding of medication administration directions or warnings. The largest item on nearly all of the labels was the pharmacy logo. The average font size was also largest for the pharmacy logo, followed by medication instructions, and drug name. Auxiliary instruction and warning stickers averaged a much smaller font size (6.5 point), too small for many older patients to see without magnification.

Additionally, the label items that were emphasized were useful to identify the pharmacy and to enhance the practice of the pharmacist, but not to help patients safely and appropriately administer medication. Typographic cues (bolding, highlighting, use of color), recommended by health literacy experts to draw attention to important text, were more commonly used for the pharmacy name or logo and other items related to the pharmacy (prescription number, refill status, and quantity). Rather than emphasizing the information patients need to take their medications safely and appropriately, current label design focuses on pharmacy brand recognition and assisting the pharmacist.

Substantial variability was also seen in the content of the labels, especially in whether or not warning/instruction stickers were used. In the reported study, between 8% and 25% of containers did not include any warning or instruction stickers. Among those that did, the variability in the content of the stickers was alarming. For the medications filled at each pharmacy, few warnings or instructions were present on more than half of the labels purchased. Among atorvastatin labels, only 42% included a warning about pregnancy, and less than 20% included directions about taking with food, taking with water, following directions precisely, and checking with a physician before starting other medications. 58% of alendronate containers included stickers instructing the patient not to lie down for 30 minutes after taking. Other warnings concerning important drug interactions and swallowing the drug whole were present on less than a third of labels. Ibuprofen containers had a broad range of warnings, but no single warning was consistently included on more than half of labels. Findings from this study suggest there is high variability in the format and content of container labels across dispensing pharmacies. More importantly, very few labels are currently designed to optimize appropriate and safe prescription medication use.

Variability also extends to how pharmacies translate physician medication instructions. In a follow-up study, researchers investigated how dosage instructions, written with common Latin abbreviations, were interpreted by various pharmacies.[40] Considerable differences were noted (see Table 2). Among the 85 labels evaluated, dose frequency was omitted on 6% of instructions ("Take 1 tablet for cholesterol").[40] Administration timing was explicitly stated on only 2% of instructions ("in the morning"). All four prescriptions noted earlier were written with an indication, yet pharmacies transcribed this onto 38% of labels. The prescription for alendronate stated to not lie down for at least 30 minutes after taking; this was transcribed with 50% of instructions. A total of 27% of the translated instructions had a Lexile reading grade level above a high school level.[23]

TABLE 2 Physician-Written Prescriptions and Pharmacy Interpretations

Prescription	Examples of Pharmacy "Sig" Interpretations

Lipitor 10 mg tabs
Take one tab QD
Dispense #30
Indication: for high
  cholesterol
No refills
	"Take one tablet daily."
	"Take 1 tablet by mouth for high cholesterol."
	"Take one (1) tablet(s) by mouth once a day."
	"Take one tablet by mouth every day for high
	  cholesterol."

Fosamax 5 mg tabs
Take one tab QD
Dispense #30
Indication: osteoporosis
  prevention
Do not lie down for at least
  30 minutes
	"Take 1 tablet by mouth daily."
	"Take one tablet by mouth every day for osteoporosis
	  prevention. Do not lie down for at least 30 minutes
	  after taking."
	"Take 1 tablet every day, 30 minutes before breakfast
	  with a glass of water. Do not lie down."
	"Take one tablet every day."

Bactrim DS tabs Take one tab BID Dispense #6 Indication: UTI No refills	"Take one tablet by mouth twice daily for UTI." "Take one tablet by mouth twice daily for urinary tract infection." "Take 1 tablet by mouth 2 times a day." "Take 1 tablet twice daily for 3 days."

Ibuprofen 200 mg tabs
Take 1-2 tabs TID PRN pain
Dispense #30
No refills
	"Take 1 to 2 tablets by mouth as needed for pain."
	"Take 1 to 2 tablets by mouth three times daily as
	  needed for pain."
	"Take 1 to 2 tablets by mouth as needed for pain
	  ** Not to exceed 4 times a day."
	"Take 1 to 2 tablets 3 times a day as needed for pain."

Health Information Technology

Tremendous advances have been made in the use of health information systems that support the prescribing and dispensing of medication. The 2006 IOM report, *The Future of Drug Safety*, directs attention to e-prescribing and the importance of health technologies for surveillance of errors and events but also to rapidly communicate risk information.[83] As more medical practices are incorporating electronic health records, many of these systems are now setting standard "sig" messages for prescribing medications for efficiency and patient safety purposes.[84] At the point of dispensing, pharmacy systems also have been using information systems to support drug labeling. This includes default standards for translating prescriber instructions and including auxiliary warnings, with set parameters for label content and format.[85,86] Currently, the Agency for Healthcare Research and Quality (AHRQ), Center for Medicare and Medicaid Studies (CMS), and National Coalition for Prescription Drug Programs have been working to develop a finite list of standard, codified "sig" lines to improve care and efficiency specifically for electronic prescribing practices.[87] A major problem that has been recognized by these organizations is the discordance between the uniform practices being developed through electronic health records at the point of prescribing and those systems in place within a majority of pharmacies in the U.S. Linking the technology on both sides to ease communication and avoiding a need for interpretation at dispensing will be an essential goal for achieving a truly standard, integrated system of patient medication information.

A BRIEF HISTORY OF DRUG LABELING

The looming problem of prescription drug container labeling is best appreciated after having a basic understanding of the relevant historical events leading up to the present circumstances. Since the formal establishment of the modern Food and Drug Administration (FDA) as a regulatory agency in 1906, four recurring themes related to drug labeling are apparent. First, oversight of drug labeling has always been a focus of the FDA, and the agency's role has gradually evolved with expanding regulatory power. Second, labeling for prescription-only medicines, in particular, is based on the assumption that physicians and other prescribers adequately communicate medication instructions to patients. Third, FDA-issued requirements for prescription drug container labeling practices are exceptionally vague. Finally, container labels for prescription-only medicines are primarily governed at the state level, and most states offer minimal guidance.

Early Attention to Drug Labeling

Instructional labels attached to vials containing the various medicines available have been in existence for centuries. Prior to the turn of the 20th century, drug container labels were designed for physician-pharmacist communication; they contained minimal content typically written in Latin abbreviations.[88] The United States Pharmacopeia (USP) was formed in 1820 to create a system of standards that would ensure quality control and drug safety. At that time, only 217 drugs met the criteria for inclusion as "most fully established and fully understood."[89] With the few possible exceptions of certain state regulations, there were no laws in place governing what could or could not be stated on the container label.[88] The Pure Food and Drugs Act of 1906 was the beginning of many federal legisla-

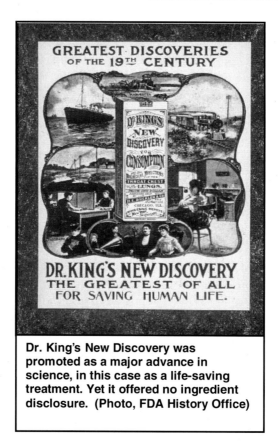

Dr. King's New Discovery was promoted as a major advance in science, in this case as a life-saving treatment. Yet it offered no ingredient disclosure. (Photo, FDA History Office)

tive responses to promote accurate and safe practices in the labeling and marketing of drugs.

The federal government response was warranted by an increasing incidence of consumer reports and investigations of patent or "quack" medicines. Many widely-used products were ineffective, addictive, or even lethal.[88] This new law focused on the regulation of product labeling rather than pre-market approval. The passage of the Pure Food and Drugs Act marked the beginning of the modern era of the FDA, and with this legislation came the beginning of a limited set of federal labeling standards. Specifically, drugs defined with standards of strength, quality and purity in the USP could not be sold in any other condition unless the variations from the standards were plainly stated on the label.[88] The new law required the contents and quantity of food and drug products be clearly identified on the label attached to the container or package. Drug labels could not be false or misleading, and the presence and amount of eleven dangerous ingredients, including alcohol, heroin, and cocaine, had to be listed on the label.[88]

What follows throughout the early decades of the 20th century is a pattern of extending federal regulatory oversight for drugs, with two distinct classifications now emerging: over-the-counter and prescription-only. This was primarily driven by a growing number of cases of unintentional drug addiction and harm. The Harrison Narcotics Act of 1914 required pharmacies to be licensed (at a cost) to dispense narcotics, and for these drugs to require a physician prescription.[90] Prior to this time, pharmacists usually followed physician recommendations and any pertinent state laws concerning dispensing practices. Problems began to emerge when physicians complained about the ability of pharmacists to dispense refills to patients for prescribed medicines without the authorization of the physician. The Harrison Act initiated the early distinction in federal statutes between the modern classifications of prescription and over-the-counter medicines, but only for a distinct class of drugs.

With growing concern over a new class of sulfa drugs among other new therapeutic agents, the Food, Drug, and Cosmetics Act of 1938 (FDCA) further grounded the FDA as an agent of public health, deeming many more new drugs too much of a hazard for self-medication and requiring a physician's prescription for use.[90] New labeling requirements were issued with the FDCA, requiring drug labels to explicitly state to consumers all ingredients, adequate directions for use, and to include warnings of potential dangers if not administered appropriately. With the new law, manufacturers had to submit a "New Drug Application" (NDA) before the drug would be approved by the FDA. The NDA had to include information about the drug and its safety, along with prescribing information. If a medicine had a narrow therapeutic margin with apparent risks, making it difficult to detail adequate instructions for safe use, the FDA's regulations required the drug label to include a statement restricting access by mandating that the drug be dispensed only through a physician's prescription. Specifically the following statement was to be included on the label: "To be used only by or on the prescription of a physician."[90] This is referred to as the prescription legend, which is still required on prescription medicine container labels to this day (although this statement was shortened to "Rx Only" in 2000).

Within two months of the passage of the FDCA, the FDA began to identify drugs such as the sulfas that could not be labeled for safe use directly by the patient—they would require a prescription from a physician. Labeling manufacturers were increasingly recognized as a serious problem. Drugs that were viewed as safe for over-the-counter use were marketed as prescription-only to avoid liability in the container/package

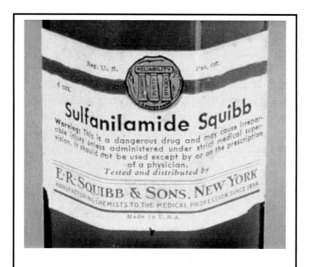

An early permutation of a prescription legend. (Photo, FDA history office)

labeling requirements for detailed instructions for use and safety warnings.[90] Laws remained unclear for prescription labeling, specifically, as the FDA assumed that physicians and pharmacists were orally communicating necessary usage directions and warnings to patients for prescribed medicines. Hence, less attention was given to the labeling on prescription drug containers or any accompanying marketing literature provided by the manufacturer. In addition, variable refill restrictions made it still possible for an individual to continue a prescription medicine, and manufacturers advertised directly to consumers to recommend their product to friends.[90] To confuse matters more, different manufacturers of the same drug often would take contradictory approaches to marketing their medicine to patients. One label might state the drug was for prescription use only, while another would be promoted for over-the-counter sale.

The Durham-Humphrey Amendment of 1951 helped put an end to some of the consumer confusion left in the wake of the FDCA, by compiling a list of medicines of the day that should be dispensed only with a physician's prescription.[90] The Amendment also established a broad outline for what constituted a prescription drug, as those medicines that were 1) habit forming, 2) toxic thereby requiring physician supervision, or

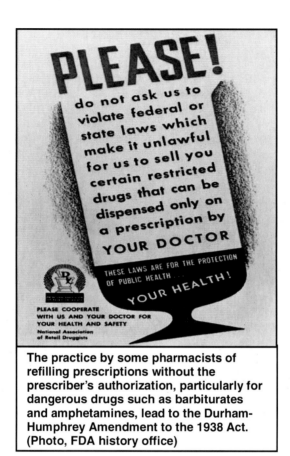

PLEASE!
do not ask us to violate federal or state laws which make it unlawful for us to sell you certain restricted drugs that can be dispensed only on a prescription by YOUR DOCTOR

THESE LAWS ARE FOR THE PROTECTION OF PUBLIC HEALTH . . . YOUR HEALTH!

PLEASE COOPERATE
WITH US AND YOUR DOCTOR FOR
YOUR HEALTH AND SAFETY
National Association
of Retail Druggists

The practice by some pharmacists of refilling prescriptions without the prescriber's authorization, particularly for dangerous drugs such as barbiturates and amphetamines, lead to the Durham-Humphrey Amendment to the 1938 Act. (Photo, FDA history office)

3) new drugs approved by the FDA with safety precautions.[90] Refills were addressed and these required physician authorization in the Durham-Humphrey Amendment, along the regulatory assumption of the FDA. Over-the-counter medicines were required to have adequate label instructions and warnings to instill safe use by the consumer, without physician consultation. However, this was not necessary for prescription-only drugs, as again it was expected access required physician consultation and information would be delivered verbally at that time. Interestingly, the Durham-Humphrey Amendment still left the ultimate determination of whether a drug would be prescription or over-the-counter to the drug manufacturer's discretion.[90]

Beyond the Bottle: The Learned Intermediary

In 1966, a pharmaceutical liability suit, Sterling Drug Inc. v. Cornish, established the physician as the "learned intermediary" with responsibility to communicate drug warnings passed on by the manufacturer to patients.[91] According to the learned intermediary doctrine, a prescription drug manufacturer fulfills its legal duty to warn a patient by adequately warning the prescribing physician. Of note, the duty to warn only the physician (and not the patient) is an exception to the general rule of law that adequate warning must reach the ultimate consumer in order for the manufacturer to avoid product liability in the case of harm. As the number of drugs labeled prescription only increased, manufacturers continued to maintain autonomy over labeling practices for these drugs. With the physician as learned intermediary, it was not viewed as necessary for prescription medicine labels to meet what constituted adequate written instructions and warnings for patients, as required under the FDCA.

With an increasingly litigious climate and society demanding more public disclosure, the need for consumer-directed prescription drug information was recognized. The Fair Packaging and Labeling Act of 1966 continued the FDA legacy of demanding honest and informative product labeling from the manufacturers themselves.[92] In line with a much earlier 1948 Supreme Court ruling in Kordel v. United States that stated supplementary materials not physically attached to the drug container could still be viewed as part of the product label, the Fair Packaging and Labeling Act mandated the inclusion of patient-directed package inserts written in lay language for all prescription drugs. This was to give patients more detailed instructions and warnings about a prescribed drug's risks and benefits, in light of container label space limitations. By the end of 1968, the first "patient package insert," or accompanying drug information sheet was issued for the asthma inhalant isoproterenol.[93] Not until 1970 with the issuance of a package insert for oral contraceptives did this requirement draw public attention.[88]

In 1979, the FDA attempted to require drug manufacturers to create patient package inserts for all prescription drugs. The FDA quickly revoked this regulation in 1981 after receiving criticism for the program by industry and health care provider organizations. In its place, drug manufacturers made a good faith agreement to "self-regulate" the industry, and generate "consumer medication information" (CMI) to be distributed with prescription medicines. In 1995, the Medication Guides program was unveiled at the FDA, which required the industry to generate yet another patient information form, for certain prescription drugs deemed to be of "serious public health concern."[88] Medication Guides are similar to the earlier patient package inserts, and are now the only consumer-directed materials for prescription drugs with explicit standards in place for their development, and to which the FDA still maintains regulatory oversight. Since 1995, more than 50 prescription medications and/or drug classes have been required to include Medication Guides. With the onset of this program, the definition of drug labeling had now expanded to include the container label, package insert, consumer medication information, and Medication Guide. The prescribing information, or "prescriber's insert," that has been required by law since 1938 for prescription-only medicines, is technically part of the label but is directed to the physician rather than the patient.

In 1997, The Keystone Dialogue, initiated by the Department of Health and Human Services and including the FDA, pharmacist associations, and the National Association of Boards of Pharmacy, was charged with developing an action plan for improving drug labeling. Recommendations targeted improvements in the reading ease of consumer medication information in order for these print materials to be accessible and useful. The published report called for consumer medication information to be written at a sixth to eighth grade level and for improved format and organization.[75] These were recommendations only, as a review of FDA-approved materials a decade later found little improvement in the quality of patient information.

The most recent labeling effort by the FDA to ensure patient understanding of appropriate prescription drug use was the June 30, 2006 revision of 21 CFR 201.56 and 201.57, "Requirements on Content and Format of Labeling for Human Prescription Drug and Biological Products." While the new law had the patient in mind, its provisions reflect the powerful role of the learned intermediary in providing essential information to the ultimate medication consumer. Revisions specifically targeted modifications to the prescriber's insert label directed to physicians. According to the new law, all inserts must contain a Highlights section summarizing drug benefits and risks, as well as a table of contents. Another new section, Patient Counseling Information, is also now included in inserts to help summarize for physicians what information about a particular drug should be conveyed to patients. This was the first change to the package insert in 25 years. However, the package insert is aimed at educating physicians rather than patients, and these changes will likely offer little relief to patients when they pick up their prescriptions at the pharmacy.[94]

The Modern Drug Container Label: Contents and Oversight

Under 21 CFR 201 of the FDCA, the FDA now requires the following information be present on the prescription drug container label: drug name, pharmacy name and address, serial/lot number of the prescription, prescribing physician name, patient name, and instructions for use.

State boards of pharmacy may impart their own additional standards for container label content and format. To date, only minimal regulations have been added by states, although enough to require national pharmacy chains to generate 31 different label styles across the 50 states.

Without explicit FDA regulatory guidance, it still remains unclear what constitutes "adequate" label instructions and warnings according to the FDCA for the more than 13,000 FDA-approved prescription medicines in use today. With the recent dominance of direct-to-consumer advertising and the 1999 ruling in Perez v. Wyeth Laboratories, Inc., the pharmaceutical industry has had to assume greater liability to directly warn consumers, beyond the learned intermediary, of any potential risks associated with using a particular medicine.[91] Such risks have usually been conveyed through the prescriber's insert (for providers) and CMI (for patients), and not directly on the container label, due to space issues.

With limited space on the primary container labels which detail dosage/use instructions, auxiliary "warning" stickers had been included with bottles as early as the late 1950s. These secondary container labels provided special instructions and precautions, often given orally to patients by the pharmacist, to support safe patient administration. However, no regulations have existed regarding the use of these auxiliary stickers either. Despite the potential value of these stickers, the accuracy of the specific instructional and/or precautionary messages has not been confirmed through any systematic process derived in pharmacological evidence.

SETTING STANDARDS:
AN EVIDENCE-BASED DRUG CONTAINER LABEL

While limited, there is evidence available to detail "best practices" for improving dosage/usage instructions written by the prescribing physician, and the format and content of prescription medication container labels designed by the dispensing pharmacy.[95] Perhaps most importantly, the use of standard and more explicit dosage/usage instructions can improve patients' functional understanding of how and when to take a medicine (i.e., take two tablets by mouth twice daily vs. take 4 tablets a day vs. take 2 tablets in the morning, and take 2 tablets in the evening).[22] Shrank and colleagues summarized known evidence for best practices in labeling format and content, such as: increasing font size, using clear and simple language, using headers, and placing a more appropriate emphasis on organizing label content around what is most important for patients (i.e., drug name, dose, dosage/usage instructions, patient name, doctor name, quantity, refill information) instead of the provider content (i.e., pharmacy name/logo, phone number, national drug code number).[95]

The field of health literacy also offers appropriate recommendations on how best to present print medication information to lower literate audiences. For instance, sans serif font should be used, avoidance of all capital letters for words and phrases, and using numbers instead of the text equivalent (i.e., 2 instead of "two").[22,95] When possible, text should be as large as 12 point font to display patient dosage/usage instructions. Icons for drug warnings have previously been found to be confusing for many older patients and those with limited literacy skills, and should be minimized in practice. A complete list of evidence-based, recommended standards for format, content, and instruction is detailed in Table 3.

TABLE 3 Description of Standards for an Enhanced Rx Container Label

Proposed Standard	Description
1. Use explicit text to describe dosage/interval in instructions.	Dosage/usage instructions must clearly separate dose from interval, and provide the explicit frequency of the drug (i.e. "take 4 tablets each day. Take 2 tablets in the morning, and 2 tablets in the evening" vs. "take two tablets by mouth twice daily"). These explicit dose/use instructions will be standardized by the pharmacy to avoid physician variability for the same dose frequency.
2. Use a universal medication schedule (UMS) to convey and simplify dosage/use instructions.	A universal medication schedule ("UMS") can help patients identify and support the explicit text dosage/usage instructions, following a familiar format to cue patients (i.e. a pill organizer external aid; with standard intervals for taking medicines: breakfast, lunch, dinner, bedtime).
3. Organize label in a patient-centered manner.	Patient-directed information must be organized in a way that best reflects how most patients seek out and understand medicine instructions. Patient-directed content will be at the top of the label, while provider-directed content will be placed at the bottom of the label. Drug name and specific dosage/usage instructions will be placed in greatest prominence.
4. Include distinguish-able front and back sides to the label.	The Rx container label should have two distinct sides—a front (primary) and back (auxiliary) side on the bottle. The primary label will contain patient information (drug name, dose, dosage/usage instructions, patient name, doctor name, quantity, refill information) and provider content (pharmacy name/logo, phone number, national drug code #). The back should contain all appropriate warning and instruction messages and icons, supplanting the use of stickers.

continued

TABLE 3 Continued

Proposed Standard	Description
5. When possible, include indication for use.	While Rx approval status and confidentiality may limit inclusion of indications for use, prior studies suggest this is very helpful to patients.
6. Simplify language, avoiding unfamiliar words/medical jargon.	Language on the label, will avoid the use of unclarified medical jargon, and common terms and sentences will be used only. While readability formulas and software are not recommended for short excerpts of text such as what is included on Rx labels, the principles established by the Suitability Assessment of Materials by Doak, Doak, and Root for maintaining simple language can guide the simplification process. Feedback should also be sought from consumers.
7. Improve typography, use larger, sans serif font.	A standard for minimum font size (12 pt) will be set for patient name, drug name, and specific dosage-usage instructions (both in text and in matrix). Health literacy and adult education researchers recommend the use of Sans-Serif font (i.e. Arial) to more clearly present print text information to new adult learners. Patient information on front and back labels will be 12 pt font. Use of all capital letters should be avoided; the first letter of words in text will be capitalized only.
8. When applicable, use numeric vs. alphabet characters.	Our recent research efforts (see Section C), and a prior study, provide evidence that presenting numbers instead of the text equivalent (i.e. 2 vs. two) was more helpful to patients for understanding and more rapidly processing dosage/usage instructions.
9. Use typographic cues (bolding and highlighting) for patient content only.	Bolding and highlighting will be used for patient-centered information only. Drug name and dose will be highlighted, dosage/usage instructions bolded.
10. Use horizontal text only.	Several national pharmacy chains place text for warning and instruction messages vertical to the Rx label; requiring the patient to turn the bottle to read. This may create further difficulty among older adults. Only include horizontal text on the label.
11. Use a standard icon system for signaling and organizing auxiliary warnings and instructions.	Work towards a standard set of icons, or consider a single icon to flag patients that a warning exists for the prescribed medicine. Warnings will use 12 point font.

Current FDA Over-The-Counter (OTC) product labeling standards may provide additional guidance to future strategies to be taken with prescription medications. OTC products, such as "Drug Facts," have already been developed with health literacy considerations in mind, utilize a standard format, and have been marketed to the public, increasing their familiarity and usability. While not all OTC labeling standards are applicable for prescription medicines, patients would likely benefit from a more familiar and consistent format, especially if this could extend to dosage/usage instructions.

SPECIFIC REPORT FINDINGS

Ideally, medication labeling should be viewed as a system of information, with key components communicated to the prescriber, the dispenser, and ultimately to patients. The work of this group has used the lens of health literacy to target patients' critical need for clear and concise prescription medication instructions to support safe and effective use. Based on the evidence and potential impact for reducing confusion that may lead to medication error, standardization of the container label's content and format, including dosage instructions, is proposed as a primary evidence-based finding that the committee viewed as necessary for resolving the current prescription labeling problem. It is anticipated that several measures will be required to address the development of low literacy-appropriate patient information leaflets and Medication Guides, and provider education and training programs to increase medication counseling and best practices for writing prescriptions.

The findings of this report support the exploration into a standard label format that may potentially include set key intervals (i.e., morning, noon, evening, bedtime) that can most precisely identify dose frequency. Currently, preliminary research activities are under way by members of the committee to investigate the efficacy of a matrix visual aid on the container label to improve patient comprehension of dosage instructions. However, before this or any other standards can be recommended, perspectives from pharmacology, pharmacy and from prescribing clinicians should be sought. More research is needed to support future actions to be taken with regard to prescription medication labeling, and all modifications to the existing labeling format should be properly evaluated.

The Committee concluded with the following findings:

1. Inadequate patient understanding of prescription medication instructions and warnings is prevalent and a significant safety concern. Health literacy research has highlighted the high prevalence of patient misunderstanding of dosage instructions and auxiliary warn-

ings placed on Rx container labels. The elderly, those with limited literacy, and individuals managing multiple medication regimens are at greater risk for misinterpreting prescription instructions.

2. Lack of universal standards and regulations for medication labeling is a "root cause" for medication error. More than a third of all reported adverse drug events occur in ambulatory care settings, where patients primarily assume quality control over prescription medication administration. Patient misuse is a common occurrence, and the clarity and complexity of medication dose/use instructions varies greatly by dispensing pharmacy. State and federal agencies involved in consumer medication information and labeling are not united in efforts to provide regulatory guidance.

3. An evidence-based set of practices should guide all label content and format. A major problem for prescription drug labeling relates to content inclusion. Efforts need to be directed at minimizing information placed on the label container, particularly auxiliary instructions supporting the safe use of the product. Only warnings and instructions that are supported by pharmacological evidence, or that are otherwise thought to significantly aid the patient in self-administration should be placed on the label. If a warning or instruction message is to be recommended for a specified drug to be on the container label, then it should be required. This would limit the existing variability between and within pharmacies.

4. Instructions for use on the container label are especially important for patients and should be written in the most clear, concise manner. Language should be standardized to improve patient understanding for safe and effective use. Variability and confusion regarding prescription drug label dosage/usage instructions is especially problematic. While auxiliary warning and instructions may vary by pharmacy, the actual instructions for dosage and use for a medicine will often vary by prescribing physician. Explicit instructions that segregate dose (number of pills to be taken at one time) from frequency (number of times per day) are more helpful to patients. Standardized, evidence-based dosage/usage instructions with limited variability would provide patients with more useful information, and offer improved drug safety for patients. A universal medication schedule would further simplify medication-taking behavior.

5. Drug labeling should be viewed as an integrated system of patient information. Improvements are needed beyond the container label, and other sources of consumer medication information should be targeted. Consumer-directed materials that accompany the pill bottle container currently do not meet acceptable standards set for the design of health information for patients with limited literacy skills.

Medication Guides, patient information leaflets, and other supplementary sources of medication information should follow the same patient-oriented schema for presenting content as the container label, and be simplified following current health literacy principles. Patients need to be involved in the re-design of these materials, and considerations of re-design should focus on all the components of the label as a system of information.

6. Health care providers are not adequately communicating to patients, either orally or in print, for prescribed medicines. More training is needed to promote best practices for writing prescriptions and counseling patients. Physicians, nurses, physician assistants and pharmacists have previously been reported as missing opportunities to adequately counsel patients on how to administer prescribed regimens. While recent FDA actions mandate content in the package insert to aid providers on what to convey to patients about specified medicines, additional training and quality improvement efforts are needed to ensure the occurrence of these practices.

7. Research support is necessary to advance the science of drug labeling and identify "best practices" for patient medication information. Ultimately, funds should be allocated to support research that can systematically review the scientific evidence and detail the necessary content for inclusion on prescription container warning labels and supplementary patient medication information materials. Likewise, health services and human factors research is needed to test new labeling strategies that incorporate known "best practices" and determine whether the changes can improve patient understanding, behaviors, and even health outcomes.

CONCLUSION

The ACPF Medication Labeling Technical Advisory Board has proposed several changes for prescription drug labeling, perhaps most notable being that dosage/usage instructions on the container label be a critical and primary focus for establishing clear standards. The importance of the container label should be reiterated as the most tangible and repeatedly used source of prescription drug instructions for use. In fact, it may be the "last line" of informational support on how and when to take a prescribed medicine. The Advisory Board agreed that prescription medication labeling should be viewed as a system of information, and additional efforts must also seek to standardize and improve labeling beyond the primary prescription container label.

It is anticipated that this report will engage policymakers, researchers, and clinicians to work toward an integrated and standard system of patient medication information. The IOM report *Preventing Medication Errors* issued a call to action to improve patient-directed medication information, including labeling and provider-patient communication. To go one step beyond the report, an agenda should be detailed that targets the prescription drug container label, and then works to integrate other formal information sources. Lessons from both the field of health literacy and human factors design should be observed. Above all, lessons from the field of health literacy underscore the need for this work to be done with patients as partners in the process, ensuring the best deliverables possible.

REFERENCES

1. Institute of Medicine. To err is human: Building a safer health system. Kohn L, Corrigan J, Donaldson M, editors. Washington, D.C.: National Academy Press; 2000.
2. Altman DE, Clancy C, Blendon RJ. Improving patient safety—five years after the IOM report. N Engl J Med 2004; 351: 2041-3.
3. Blendon RJ, DesRoches CM, Brodie M, Benson JM, Rosen AB, Schneider E, et al. Views of practicing physicians and the public on medical errors. N Engl J Med. 2002; 347: 1933-40.
4. Vincent C. Understanding and responding to adverse events. N Engl J Med 2003; 348:1051-6.
5. Leape LL. Reporting of adverse events. N Engl J Med 2002; 347:1633-8.
6. Elder NC, Dovey SM. Classification of medical errors and preventable adverse events in primary care: a synthesis of the literature. J Fam Pract 2002; 51: 927-32.
7. Gandhi TK, Weingart SN, Borus J, Seger AC, Peterson J, Burdick E, et al. Adverse drug events in ambulatory care. N Engl J Med 2003; 348: 1556-1564.
8. Gurwitz JH, Field TS, Harrold LR, Rothschild J, Debellis K, Seger A, et al. Incidence and preventability of adverse drug events among older persons in the ambulatory setting. JAMA 2003; 289: 1107-1116.
9. Forster AJ, Murff HJ, Peterson JF, Gandhi TK, Bates DW. The incidence and severity of adverse events affecting patients after discharge from the hospital. Ann Intern Med 2003;138: 161-7.
10. Hammons T, Piland NF, Small SD, Hatlie MJ, Burstin HR. Ambulatory patient safety. What we know and need to know. J Ambul Care Manage 2003; 26:63-82.
11. Gandhi TK, Burstin HR, Cook EF, et al. Drug complications in outpatients. J Gen Intern Med 2000; 15:149-54.
12. Dovey SM, Meyers DS, Phillips RL, et al. A preliminary taxonomy of medical errors in family practice. Qual Saf Health Care 2002; 11:233-8.
13. Plews-Ogan ML, Nadkarni MM, Forren S, Leon D, White D, Marineau D, et al. Patient safety in the ambulatory setting. A clinician-based approach. J Gen Intern Med 2004; 19:719-25.
14. Budnitz DS, Layde PM. Outpatient drug safety: new steps in an old direction. Pharmacoepidemiol Drug Saf; 2007; 16: (2) 160.
15. Bates DW, Spell N, Cullen D, Burdick E, Laird N, Peterson L, et al. The costs of adverse drug events in hospitalized patients. JAMA 1997; 277:307-311.
16. Poon EG, Cina JL, Churchill W, Patel N, Featherstone E, Rothschild JM. Medication dispensing errors and potential adverse drug events before and after implementing bar code technology in the pharmacy. Ann Intern Med 2006; 145:426-34.

17. Barker KN, Flynn EA, Pepper GA, Bates DW, Mikeal RL. Medication errors observed in 36 health care facilities. Arch Intern Med 2002;162:1897-903.

18. Barker KN, Mikeal RL, Pearson RE, Illig NA, Morse ML. Medication errors in nursing homes and small hospitals. Am J Hosp Pharm 1982; 39: 987-91.

19. Gurwitz JH, Field TS, Judge J, Rochon P, Harrold LR, Cadoret C, et al. The incidence of adverse drug events in two large academic long-term care facilities. Am J Med 2005; 118:251-8.

20. Institute of Medicine. Preventing Medication Errors. Aspden P, Wolcott J, Bootman L, Cronenwett LR (eds). Washington D.C., National Academy Press, 2006.

21. Medical Expenditure Panel Survey [on-line]. Available at http://www.meps.ahrq.gov. Accessed January 3, 2007.

22. Davis TC, Wolf MS, Bass PF, Tilson H, Neuberger M, Parker RM. Literacy and misunderstanding of prescription drug labels. Ann Intern Med 2006; 145: 887-94.

23. Davis TC, Wolf MS, Bass PF, Middlebrooks M, Kennan E, Baker DW, Bennett CL, Durazo-Arvizu R, Savory S, Parker RM. Low literacy impairs comprehension of prescription drug warning labels. J Gen Intern Med 2006; 21: 847-851.

24. Institute of Medicine. Health Literacy: A prescription to end confusion. Nielsen-Bohlman L, Panzer A, Kindig DA, editors. Washington, D.C., National Academy Press 2004.

25. Kutner M, Greenberg E, Baer J. A first look at the literacy of America's adults in the 21st century. National Center for Education Statistics, U.S. Department of Education, 2005.

26. Baker DW. The meaning and the measure of health literacy. J Gen Intern Med 2006: 21: 878-883.

27. DeWalt DA, Pignone MP. Reading is fundamental: the relationship between literacy and health. Arch Intern Med 2005 Sep 26;165(17):1943-4.

28. Rudd RE, Renzulli D, Pereira A, Daltroy L. Literacy demands in health care settings: the patient perspective, in Schwartzberg JG, VanGeest JB, Wang CC (eds.): Understanding health literacy: Implications for medicine and public health. Chicago, IL, AMA Press, 2004, pp. 69-84.

29. Castro CM, Wilson C, Schillinger D. Babel- should this Babble? Babble: Physicians' use of unclarified medical jargon with patients who have type 2 diabetes and limited health literacy. In press- still in press?, Am J Health Behav 2007.

30. Kutner, M., Greenberg, E., Jin, Y., & Paulsen, C. (2006). The Health Literacy of America's Adults: Results from the 2003 National Assessment of Adult Literacy (NCES 2006-483). U.S. Department of Education. Washington, DC: National Center for Education Statistics.

31. Tarn DM, Heritage J, Paterniti DA, Hays RD, Kravitz RL, Wenger NS. Physician communication when prescribing new medications. Arch Intern Med 2006; 166:1855-62.

32. Morris LA, Tabak ER, Gondel K. Counseling patients about prescribed medications: 12-year trend. Med Care 1997; 35: 996-1007.

33. Metlay JP, Cohen A, Polsky D, Kimmel SE, Koppel R, Hennessy S. Medication safety in older adults: home-based practice patterns. J Am Geriatr Soc 2005; 53: 976-982.

34. Sleath B, Roter D, Chewning B, et al. Asking questions about medication: analysis of physician-patient interactions and physician perceptions. Med Care 1999; 37:1169-73.

35. Stevenson FA, Cox K, Britten N, et al. A systematic review of the research on communication between patients and health care professionals about medicines: the consequences for concordance. Health Expect 2004; 7: 235-45.

36. Schillinger D, Piette J, Grumbach K, Wang F, et al. Closing the loop: Physician communication with diabetic patients who have low health literacy. Arch Intern Med 2003:163: 83-90.

37. Weiss BD, Coyne C, and Michielutte, R., et al. Communicating with patients who have limited literacy skills: Consensus statement from the National Work Group on Literacy and Health. J Family Practice 1998, 46:168-176.

38. Davis TC, Williams MV, Branch, Jr., WT, Green KW. Explaining illness to patients with limited literacy. In: Whaley, Bryan B. (ed.). Explaining Illness: Research, Theory, and Strategies. Mahway, New Jersey: Larence Erlbaum Associates, 2000: 123-146.

39. Dunn EB, Wolfe JJ. Let go of Latin! Vet Hum Toxicol 2001; 43: 235-6.

40. Wolf MS, Shrank WH, Choudry NK, Agnew-Blais J, Parker RM, Shekelle P. Variability in Pharmacy Interpretations of Physician Prescriptions. Under review, Journal of General Internal Medicine.

41. Wallace LS, Roskos SE, Weiss BD. Readability characteristics of consumer medication information for asthma inhalation devices. J Asthma 2006; 43:375-8.

42. Wallace LS, Rogers ES, Turner LW, Keenum AJ, Weiss BD. Suitability of written supplemental materials available on the Internet for nonprescription medications. Am J Health Syst Pharm 2006 Jan 1;63(1):71-8.

43. Kang E, Fields HW, Cornett S, Beck FM. An evaluation of pediatric dental patient education materials using contemporary health literacy measures. Pediatr Dent 2005; 27: 409-13.

44. Kaphingst KA, Zanfini CJ, Emmons KM. Accessibility of web sites containing colorectal cancer information to adults with limited literacy. Cancer Causes Control 2006; 17: 147-51.

45. Weintraub D, Maliski SL, Fink A, Choe S, Litwin MS. Suitability of prostate cancer education materials: applying a standardized assessment tool to currently available materials. Patient Educ Couns 2004; 55:275-80.

46. Wolf MS, Davis TC, Shrank W, Neuberger M, Parker RM. A critical review of FDA-approved Medication Guides. Pat Educ Counsel 2006; 62: 316-22.

47. Peterson G, Aslani P, Williams KA. How do consumers search for and appraise information on medicines on the Internet? A qualitative study using focus groups. J Med Internet Res 2003; 5: e33.

48. Batchlor E, Laouri M. Pharmaceutical promotion, advertising, and consumers. Health Aff 2003; Jan-Jun Suppl: W3-109-11.

49. Rosenthal MB, Berndt ER, Donohue JM, Frank RG, Epstein AM. Promotion of prescription drugs to consumers. N Engl J Med 2002; 346: 498-505.

50. Wolf MS, Davis TC, Arozullah A, Penn R, Arnold C, Bennett CL. Relationship between literacy and HIV treatment knowledge among individuals enrolled in HAART regimens. AIDS Care 2005; 17: 863-873.

51. Wolf MS, Davis TC, Cross JT, Marin E, Green KM, Bennett CL. Health literacy and patient knowledge in a Southern U.S. HIV clinic. Int J STD AIDS 2004; 15: 747-752.

52. Davis TC, Fredrickson DD, Potter L, Brouillette R, Bocchini AC, Williams MV, Parker RM. Patient understanding and use of oral contraceptive pills in a southern public health family planning clinic. South Med J 2006; 99:713-8.

53. Dowse R, Ehlers MS. The influence of education on the interpretation of pharmaceutical pictograms for communicating medicine instructions. Intern J Pharm Pract 2003; 11: 11-18.

54. Insel K, Morrow D, Brewer B, Figueredo A. Executive function, working memory, and medication adherence among older adults. J Gerontol B Psychol Sci Soc Sci 2006: 61: 102-107.

55. Stilley CS, Sereika S, Muldoon MF, Ryan CM, Dunbar-Jacob J. Psychological and cognitive function: predictors of adherence with cholesterol lowering treatment. Ann Behav Med 2004: 27: 117-124.

56. Gazmararian JA, Kripalani S, Miller MJ, Echt KV, Ren J, Rask K. Factors associated with medication refill adherence in cardiovascular-related diseases: a focus on health literacy. J Gen Intern Med 2006; 21:1215-1221.

57. Kalichman SC, Ramachandran B, Catz S. Adherence to combination antiretroviral therapies in HIV patients of low health literacy. J Gen Intern Med 1999; 14:267-273.

58. Chia LR, Schlenk EA, Dunbar-Jacob J. Effect of personal and cultural beliefs on medication adherence in the elderly. Drugs Aging 2006; 23:191-202.

59. Brown M, Frost R, Ko Y, Woosley R. Diagramming patients' views of root causes of adverse drug events in ambulatory care: an online tool for planning educational research. Pat Educ Counsel 2006; 62: 302-315.

60. Wolf MS, Davis TC, Bass PF, Tilson H, Parker RM. Misunderstanding prescription drug warning labels among patients with low literacy. Am J Health System Pharm 2006; 63: 1048-55.

61. National Council on Patient Information and Education (NCPIE) [on-line]. Available at: http://www.talkaboutrx.org/. Accessed August 15, 2007.

62. Morrow DG, Leirer VO, Sheikh J. Adherence and medication instructions: review and recommendations. J Am Geriatric Soc 1988; 36: 1147-1160.

63. Park DC, Jones TR. Medication adherence and aging. In Fisk AD, Rogers WA (eds) Handbook of Human Factors and the Older Adult (pp. 257-287), San Diego, CA: Academic Press, 1997.

64. Rice GE, Okun MA. Older readers' processing of medical information that contradicts their beliefs. J Gerontol: Psych Sci 1994: 49: 119-128.

65. Gien L, Anderson JA. Medication and the elderly: a review. J Geriatric Drug Ther 1989; 4: 59-89.

66. Park DC, Morrell RW, Frieske D, Blackburn AB, Birchmore. Cognitive factors and the use of over-the-counter medication organizers by arthritis patients. Human Factors 1991; 33: 57-67.

67. Park DC, Morrell RW, Frieske D, Kincaid D. Medication adherence behaviors in older adults: effects of external cognitive supports. Psychol & Aging 1992; 7: 252-256.

68. Morrow DG. Elder's schema for taking medication: implications for instructional design. J Gerontol Psych Sci 1991; 46: 378-385.

69. Prescription drug product labeling: FDA Medication Guide requirements. Final rule. Fed Regist 1998; 63: 66378-400.

70. Medication Guides for Prescription Drug Products. Code of Federal Regulations 2004 ed. Title 21; Pt 208: 111-114.

71. Status of Useful Written Prescription Drug Information for Patients; Docket No 00N-0352. Federal Register 65 (28 April 2000): 7022.

72. American Pharmaceutical Association. Committee Policy Report on Health Literacy 2001-2002.

73. American Society of Health-System Pharmacists. ASHP Guidelines on Pharmacist-Conducted Patient Education and Counseling. Medication Therapy and Patient Care: Organization and Delivery of Services-Guidelines 1997; 192-4.

74. The American Pharmaceutical Association and APhA Foundation: Pharmacy and You: www.pharmacyandyou.org.- accessed on February 28, 2007.

75. Keystone Center. 1996. The final report of the Keystone national policy dialogue on food, nutrition, and health. Keystone, CO and Washington, DC.

76. Krass I, Svarstad BL, Bultman D. Using alternative methodologies for evaluating patient medication leaflets. Patient Educ Couns 2002; 47: 29-35.

77. Gustafsson J, Kalvemark S, Nilsson G, et al. Patient information leaflets: patients' comprehension of information about interactions and contraindications. Pharm World Sci 2005; 27: 35-40.

78. Wolf MS, Davis TC, Cross JT, Marin E, Green KM, Bennett CL. Health literacy and patient knowledge in a Southern U.S. HIV clinic. Int J STD AIDS 2004; 15: 747-752.

79. Wolf MS, Williams MV, Parker RM, Parikh NS, Nowlan AW, Baker DW. Patient's shame and attitudes toward discussing the results of literacy screening. Journal of Health Communication, in press 2007.

80. Baker DW, Parker RM, Williams MV, Pitkin K, Parikh NS, Coates W, Imara M. The health care experience of patients with low literacy. Arch Fam Med 1996;5:329-34.

81. Parikh NS, Parker RM, Nurss JR, Baker DW, Williams MV. Shame and health literacy: the unspoken connection. Patient Educ Couns 1996;27:33-9.

82. Shrank WH, Agnew-Blais J, Choudry N, Wolf MS, Kesselheim A, Avorn JL, Shekelle. The variability and poor quality of medication container labels: A prescription for confusion. In press, Archives of Internal Medicine.

83. Institute of Medicine. The future of drug safety: promoting and protecting the health of the public. Baciu A, Stratton K, Burke S, editors. Washington, D.C.: National Academy Press; 2006.

84. Epic Company [on-line]. Available at http://www.epicsystems.com/Company/About. php. Accessed August 20, 2007.

85. Medi-Span [on-line]. Available at http://www.medispan.com. Accessed August 20, 2007.

86. National Council for Prescription Drug Programs [on-line] Available at http://www. ncpdp.org. Accessed August 20, 2007.

87. Electronic Prescribing Initiative eHealth Initiative. Electronic Prescribing: Toward Maximum Value and Rapid Adoption. Recommendations for optimal design and implementation to improve care, increase efficiency and reduce costs in ambulatory care. Agency for Healthcare Research and Quality (AHRQ); Washington DC, April 14, 2004.

88. Swann J. Evolution of the drug label. Food, Drug, Cosm Med Device L Digest 1998; 15: 23-31.

89. US Pharmacopeia History [on-line]. Available at http://www.usp.org/aboutUSP/ history.html. Accessed February 8, 2007.

90. Swann J. The FDA and the practice of pharmacy: prescription drug regulation before 1968, in Spillane JF, Erlen J (eds.): Federal drug control: The evolution of policy and practice. New York, NY, Haworth Press, 2004, pp 145-166.

91. Gemperli MP. Rethinking the role of the learned intermediary: the effect of direct-to-consumer advertising on litigation. JAMA 2000; 284:2241.

92. 33 Fed. Reg. 8812 (1968) (codified at 21 C.F.R. §201.305).

93. Public Law 93-608, 3 Nov. 1966, 80 U. S. Stat.

94. Avorn J, Shrank W. Highlights and a hidden hazard—the FDA's new labeling regulations. N Engl J Med. 2006 Jun 8;354(23):2409-11.

95. Shrank WH, Avorn J, Rolón C, Shekelle P. The Effect of the Content and Format of Prescription Drug Labels on Readability, Understanding and Medication Use: A Systematic Review. Ann Pharmacother. 2007 May;41(5):783-801.